Moxibustion

Ancient Healing for Modern Living

Mei Lin Zhang

Xspurts.com

A New Zealand Designed Product

Other Versions Available

Why limit yourself to just one format?

This book is now available in physical, digital, and audiobook options.

Choose the way you love to read and dive into the story today. You won't regret it!

Digital ISBN: 9781776968114
Physical ISBN: 9781776968107
Audio ISBN:

To obtain a different format of this book at a discounted price, please get in touch with us at:

http://isbn.xspurts.com/

Contents

Have Questions / Comments?

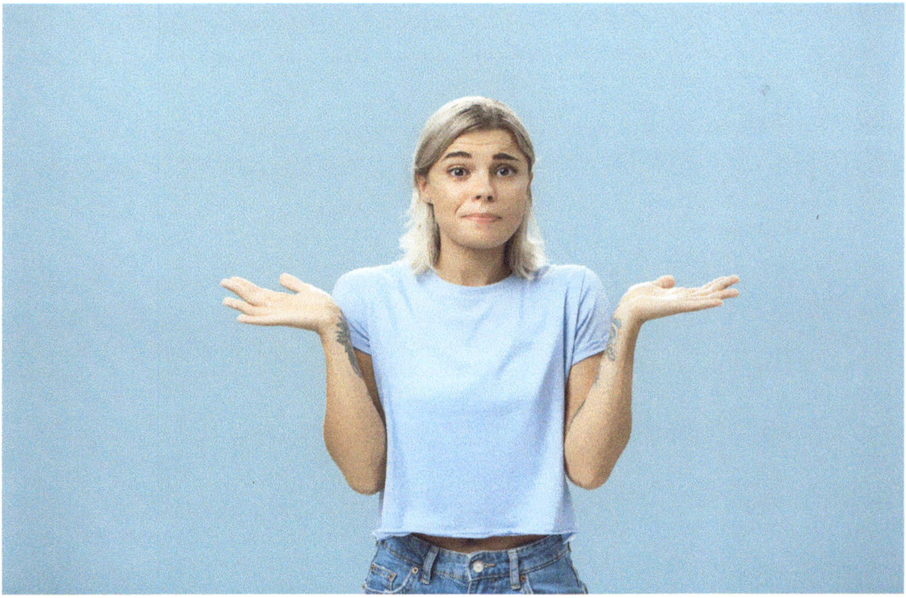

This book was designed to cover as much information as possible, but I know I have probably missed something, or some new amazing discovery has just come out.

If you notice something missing or have a question that I failed to answer, please get in touch and let me know. If I can, I will email you an answer and also update the book so others can also benefit from it.

Thanks For Being Awesome :)

Submit Your Questions / Comments At:

https://questions.xspurts.com

Get Free Stuff

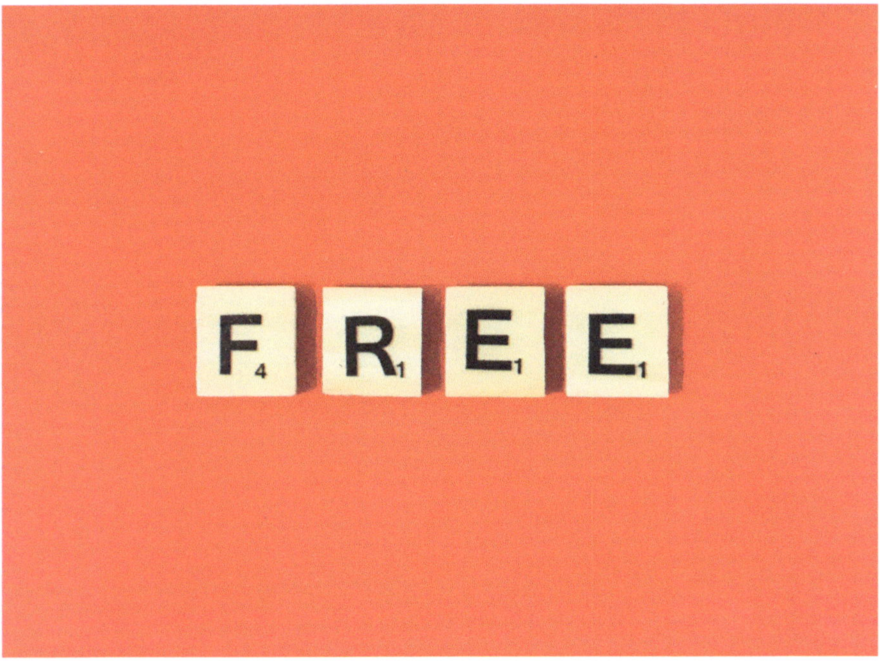

We love writing and have produced a huge number of books.

For being one of our amazing readers, we would love to offer you more books we have created, 100% free.

To claim this limited time special offer, simply go to the site below and enter your name and email address.

You will then receive loads (as we love our readers so much :) of our great books, content and audio direct to your email account, 100% free!

Get Loads of FREE Stuff at:

https://free.xspurts.com

Chapter One

Introduction to Moxibustion

Moxibustion is a traditional Chinese medicine practice that involves the burning of dried mugwort on or near specific points on the body. It is a form of heat therapy that has been used for over 2,500 years to treat a wide range of ailments and conditions.

The word "moxibustion" is derived from the Japanese words "mogusa," which means mugwort, and "shin," which means to burn. Mugwort is a plant that has been used in traditional medicine for centuries, and it is believed to have a wide range of therapeutic properties.

In moxibustion, dried mugwort is usually rolled into a stick or cone shape and then lit with a flame. The burning mugwort is then held close to the skin or placed on the skin directly, on or near specific points on the body known as acupuncture points. The heat from the burning mugwort is believed to stimulate these points and promote healing.

Moxibustion is often used in conjunction with acupuncture, which is another traditional Chinese medicine practice. Acupuncture involves the insertion of thin needles into specific points on the body, and it is believed to promote healing and alleviate pain.

1. There are two main types of moxibustion: direct and indirect. In direct moxibustion, a small amount of mugwort is placed directly on the skin and burned. This type of moxibustion can be further divided into two subtypes: scarring and non-scarring. Scarring moxibustion involves

burning the mugwort until it leaves a scar on the skin, while non-scarring moxibustion involves burning the mugwort until it is hot, but not until it causes a scar.

Indirect moxibustion involves placing a barrier between the burning mugwort and the skin, such as a slice of ginger, garlic, or salt. The heat from the burning mugwort is then transmitted through the barrier and onto the skin.

Moxibustion is believed to have a wide range of therapeutic effects. It is commonly used to treat pain, particularly chronic pain, and it is believed to be especially effective in treating musculoskeletal pain, such as back pain and arthritis. It is also used to treat digestive disorders, such as irritable bowel syndrome and constipation, and respiratory disorders, such as asthma and bronchitis. In addition, moxibustion is believed to be effective in treating menstrual cramps and other gynecological disorders, as well as depression and anxiety.

The therapeutic effects of moxibustion are believed to be due to its ability to stimulate the flow of qi, or vital energy, in the body. According to traditional Chinese medicine, qi flows through the body along pathways known as meridians. When the flow of qi is disrupted, illness and disease can occur. Moxibustion is believed to stimulate the flow of qi along these meridians, thus promoting healing and alleviating symptoms.

In addition to its therapeutic effects, moxibustion is also believed to have a number of other benefits. It is believed to strengthen the immune system, improve circulation, and promote relaxation and stress relief.

Moxibustion is generally considered to be a safe and non-invasive therapy. However, it is not suitable for everyone. People with certain conditions, such as cancer or skin conditions, may not be able to undergo moxibustion, and it should always be performed by a qualified practitioner.

History and Origins

Moxibustion is a traditional Chinese medicine practice that has been used for over 2,500 years to treat a wide range of ailments and conditions. The origins of moxibustion can be traced back to ancient China, where it was first developed as a way to promote healing and alleviate pain.

The earliest records of moxibustion date back to the Han Dynasty (206 BCE-220 CE), when it was first mentioned in the ancient Chinese medical text known as the Huangdi Neijing or Yellow Emperor's Classic of Internal Medicine. The text describes moxibustion as a method of treating illnesses by burning moxa, a substance made from dried mugwort, on or near specific points on the body.

Over the centuries, moxibustion continued to be used and refined by Chinese physicians and healers. It became a popular form of therapy in Japan and Korea, where it is known as moxa, and it eventually spread to other parts of the world as well.

One of the key figures in the development of moxibustion was a physician and scholar named Zhang Zhongjing, who lived during the Eastern Han Dynasty (25-220 CE). Zhang Zhongjing is widely considered to be one of the most important figures in the history of Chinese medicine, and his contributions to the field are still revered today.

Zhang Zhongjing is credited with developing a type of moxibustion known as "warm needling," which involves inserting an acupuncture needle into an acupuncture point and then heating the needle with a burning stick of moxa. This technique is still used today in traditional Chinese medicine.

Another important figure in the history of moxibustion was Wang Weiyi, a physician who lived during the Northern Song Dynasty (960-1127 CE). Wang Weiyi is credited with developing a system of acupuncture and moxibustion that is still used today in traditional Chinese medicine.

During the Ming Dynasty (1368-1644 CE), moxibustion became even more widely used, and it was included in the official medical texts of the time. The Ming Dynasty was a period of great cultural and scientific achievement in China, and many of the medical practices and theories developed during this time continue to be used today.

Despite its long history and widespread use, moxibustion has not always been accepted by the Western medical establishment. In the 19th century, when Western medicine began to gain popularity in China, moxibustion and other traditional medical practices were viewed as outdated and inferior to Western medicine.

However, in recent years, there has been a growing interest in traditional Chinese medicine and moxibustion in the West. Many people are turning to these ancient healing practices as a way to complement or even replace Western medical treatments.

Today, moxibustion is used to treat a wide range of conditions, including pain, digestive disorders, respiratory problems, and gynecological issues. It is often used in conjunction with acupuncture, and the two practices are believed to complement each other.

While the exact mechanisms of action of moxibustion are not yet fully understood, it is believed to work by stimulating the flow of qi, or vital energy, in the body. According to traditional Chinese medicine, when the flow of qi is disrupted, illness and disease can occur. Moxibustion is believed to stimulate the flow of qi along the meridians, thus promoting healing and alleviating symptoms.

In addition to its therapeutic effects, moxibustion is also believed to have a number of other benefits. It is believed to strengthen the immune system, improve circulation, and promote relaxation and stress relief.

Despite its long history and widespread use, there is still much that is not known about

Principles and Theory

Moxibustion is a traditional Chinese medicine practice that involves the burning of dried mugwort on or near specific points on the body. It is based on the principles and theories of traditional Chinese medicine, which views the body as a complex system of interrelated parts and energies.

According to traditional Chinese medicine, the body is governed by a vital energy called qi, which flows through the body along pathways known as meridians. When the flow of qi is disrupted or blocked, illness and disease can occur. Moxibustion is believed to stimulate the flow of qi along the meridians, thus promoting healing and alleviating symptoms.

There are several key principles and theories that underpin moxibustion, including the principles of yin and yang, the five elements, and the zang-fu organs.

The principle of yin and yang is a fundamental concept in traditional Chinese medicine. It refers to the opposing forces that govern the universe, including the body. Yin is associated with darkness, cold, and rest, while yang is associated with light, warmth, and activity. In traditional Chinese medicine, health is believed to be maintained when the balance between yin and yang is in harmony. Moxibustion is believed to help restore the balance of yin and yang in the body.

The principle of the five elements is another important concept in traditional Chinese medicine. It refers to the five elements of nature, including wood, fire, earth, metal, and water. Each element is associated with specific organs, emotions, and other aspects of the body. Moxibustion is believed to help regulate the flow of energy between these elements, thus promoting health and well-being.

The zang-fu organs are another key concept in traditional Chinese medicine. The zang organs refer to the solid organs of the body, such as the heart, liver, and kidneys, while the fu organs refer to the hollow organs, such as the stomach and intestines. Each organ is believed to have its own unique energy and function, and moxibustion is often used to stimulate or regulate these energies.

There are several theories that attempt to explain the mechanisms of action of moxibustion. One theory is that moxibustion works by increasing the production of white blood cells and other immune system components, thus strengthening the immune system and promoting healing.

Another theory is that moxibustion works by increasing blood flow and oxygenation to the affected area, thus promoting healing and reducing inflammation. Moxibustion is also believed to stimulate the production of endorphins, which are natural painkillers produced by the body.

Moxibustion is typically performed by a qualified practitioner who has undergone specialized training in traditional Chinese medicine. The practitioner will first perform a thorough examination and diagnosis of the patient's condition, taking into account factors such as the patient's medical history, symptoms, and overall health.

Once a diagnosis has been made, the practitioner will choose specific acupuncture points and apply moxibustion to these points using either direct or indirect methods. Direct moxibustion involves placing a small amount of moxa directly on the skin and lighting it, while indirect moxibustion involves using a barrier, such as ginger or salt, to prevent the moxa from coming into direct contact with the skin.

The duration and frequency of moxibustion treatments can vary depending on the patient's condition and overall health. Some patients may only require a few treatments, while others may require ongoing treatment over a longer period of time.

Different Types of Moxibustion

Moxibustion is a traditional Chinese medicine practice that involves the burning of dried mugwort on or near specific points on the body. There are several different types of moxibustion, each of which is believed to have its own unique benefits and uses.

Direct Moxibustion

1. Direct moxibustion involves placing a small amount of moxa directly on the skin and lighting it. The moxa is allowed to burn until it is extinguished or until the patient experiences a strong sensation of warmth. Direct moxibustion can be further divided into two subtypes: scarring and non-scarring.

Scarring moxibustion involves burning the moxa until it leaves a scar on the skin. This type of moxibustion is believed to be particularly effective in treating chronic conditions, such as arthritis and musculoskeletal pain.

Non-scarring moxibustion involves burning the moxa until it is hot, but not until it causes a scar. This type of moxibustion is believed to be less intense than scarring moxibustion, and it is often used to treat acute conditions, such as colds and flu.

Indirect Moxibustion

Indirect moxibustion involves placing a barrier between the moxa and the skin, such as a slice of ginger, garlic, or salt. The moxa is then placed on top of the barrier and allowed to burn until it is extinguished or until the patient experiences a strong sensation of warmth.

Indirect moxibustion is believed to be less intense than direct moxibustion, and it is often used to treat more sensitive areas of the body, such as the face and genitals. It is also believed to be more hygienic than direct moxibustion, as it reduces the risk of infection.

Needle Moxibustion

Needle moxibustion involves placing a small amount of moxa on the end of an acupuncture needle and then lighting it. The heat from the burning moxa is then transmitted through the needle and into the acupuncture point.

Needle moxibustion is believed to be particularly effective in treating chronic conditions, such as arthritis and musculoskeletal pain. It is often used in conjunction with acupuncture, and the two practices are believed to complement each other.

Warm Needle Moxibustion

Warm needle moxibustion involves inserting an acupuncture needle into an acupuncture point and then heating the needle with a burning stick of moxa. The heat from the moxa is believed to enhance the therapeutic effects of acupuncture.

Warm needle moxibustion is believed to be particularly effective in treating conditions such as digestive disorders and gynecological issues. It is also believed to be effective in promoting relaxation and reducing stress.

Infrared Moxibustion

Infrared moxibustion is a newer form of moxibustion that uses infrared light to deliver heat to the acupuncture points. Infrared moxibustion is believed to be less intense than other forms of moxibustion, and it is often used to treat more sensitive areas of the body, such as the face and genitals.

Infrared moxibustion is also believed to be more hygienic than other forms of moxibustion, as it eliminates the need for direct contact between the moxa and the skin.

Chapter Two

Tools and Materials

Moxibustion is a traditional Chinese medicine practice that involves the burning of dried mugwort on or near specific points on the body. There are several different tools and materials used in moxibustion, each of which is essential to the practice.

Moxa

The primary material used in moxibustion is moxa, a substance made from dried mugwort. Moxa can come in several different forms, including sticks, cones, and loose fibers.

Moxa is typically made by harvesting mugwort leaves and drying them in the sun. The dried leaves are then ground into a fine powder, which is shaped into sticks or cones. Some types of moxa are also made by twisting the dried leaves into loose fibers.

Moxa is believed to have a number of therapeutic benefits, including the ability to promote healing, alleviate pain, and stimulate the immune system.

Acupuncture Needles

Acupuncture needles are another essential tool used in moxibustion. Acupuncture needles are thin, sterile needles that are inserted into specific acupuncture points on the body. These needles are made from stainless steel and are typically disposable.

Acupuncture needles are often used in combination with moxibustion, particularly in the practice of warm needle moxibustion. In this technique, a small amount of moxa is placed on the end of an acupuncture needle and then lit. The heat from the burning moxa is then transmitted through the needle and into the acupuncture point.

Moxa Holders

Moxa holders are used to hold the moxa sticks or cones during moxibustion. There are several different types of moxa holders, including metal, ceramic, and bamboo.

Metal moxa holders are typically made from stainless steel and are designed to hold the moxa stick or cone at a safe distance from the skin. Ceramic moxa holders are similar to metal holders, but they are often designed with intricate patterns and designs.

Bamboo moxa holders are a traditional type of moxa holder that is still used today. They are made from bamboo and are designed to hold the moxa stick or cone close to the skin.

Moxa Burners

Moxa burners are used to burn loose moxa fibers. These burners are typically made from ceramic or metal and are designed to hold the moxa fibers while they burn.

Some moxa burners are designed to be placed on the skin, while others are designed to be held in the hand. There are also portable moxa burners that can be used on the go.

Ginger or Salt Barriers

Ginger or salt barriers are used in indirect moxibustion to prevent the moxa from coming into direct contact with the skin. These barriers are typically made from ginger or salt and are placed on the skin before the moxa is applied.

Ginger and salt barriers are believed to have additional therapeutic benefits of their own. Ginger is believed to have anti-inflammatory properties, while salt is believed to have a purifying effect on the body.

Moxa Sticks

Moxibustion is a traditional Chinese medicine practice that involves the burning of dried mugwort on or near specific points on the body. One of the most common forms of moxa is in the form of moxa sticks. Moxa sticks are made by compressing dried mugwort into a stick or cigar shape. They are an essential tool used in moxibustion and are believed to have a number of therapeutic benefits.

The Process of Making Moxa Sticks

Moxa sticks are made from dried mugwort leaves. The leaves are first harvested and then dried in the sun. Once the leaves are dry, they are ground into a fine powder. The powder is then mixed with a binding agent, typically rice flour or another type of starch. The mixture is then formed into sticks or cigars, which are left to dry.

The dried moxa sticks are then ready to be used in moxibustion. When the moxa sticks are burned, they release a fragrant smoke that is believed to have a number of therapeutic benefits.

Types of Moxa Sticks

There are several different types of moxa sticks, each of which is believed to have its own unique benefits and uses.

Pure Moxa Sticks

Pure moxa sticks are made from 100% pure dried mugwort. These sticks are believed to be the most potent form of moxa and are often used to treat chronic conditions, such as arthritis and musculoskeletal pain.

Smokeless Moxa Sticks

Smokeless moxa sticks are a newer form of moxa that is designed to reduce the amount of smoke produced during moxibustion. These sticks are made from a mixture of dried mugwort and other herbs, such as sage or lavender. The addition of these herbs is believed to reduce the amount of smoke produced while still maintaining the therapeutic benefits of moxibustion.

Charcoal Moxa Sticks

Charcoal moxa sticks are made by adding a small amount of charcoal powder to the dried mugwort mixture. The charcoal is believed to enhance the therapeutic effects of moxibustion by increasing the heat and reducing the amount of smoke produced.

Wormwood and Mugwort Moxa Sticks

Wormwood and mugwort moxa sticks are made by combining dried wormwood and mugwort. Wormwood is believed to have additional therapeutic benefits, including the ability to kill parasites and promote digestion.

How Moxa Sticks are Used in Moxibustion

Moxa sticks are typically used in direct moxibustion, which involves placing a small amount of moxa directly on the skin and lighting it. The moxa is allowed to burn until it is extinguished or until the patient experiences a strong sensation of warmth.

Moxa sticks can also be used in indirect moxibustion, which involves using a barrier, such as ginger or salt, to prevent the moxa from coming into direct contact with the skin. In indirect moxibustion, the moxa stick is placed on top of the barrier and allowed to burn until it is extinguished or until the patient experiences a strong sensation of warmth.

Benefits of Moxa Sticks

Moxa sticks are believed to have a number of therapeutic benefits, including the ability to promote healing, alleviate pain, and stimulate the immune system. Moxa sticks are often used to treat conditions such as arthritis, musculoskeletal pain, digestive disorders, and gynecological issues.

Moxa sticks are also believed to promote relaxation and reduce stress. The fragrant smoke produced by burning moxa sticks is believed to have a calming effect on the body and mind.

Moxa Cones

Moxibustion is a traditional Chinese medicine practice that involves the burning of dried mugwort on or near specific points on the body. One of the most common forms of moxa is in the form of moxa cones. Moxa cones are made by compressing dried mugwort into a cone shape. They are an essential tool used in moxibustion and are believed to have a number of therapeutic benefits.

The Process of Making Moxa Cones

Moxa cones are made from dried mugwort leaves. The leaves are first harvested and then dried in the sun. Once the leaves are dry, they are ground into a fine powder. The powder is then mixed with a binding agent, typically rice flour or another type of starch. The mixture is then formed into cones, which are left to dry.

The dried moxa cones are then ready to be used in moxibustion. When the moxa cones are burned, they release a fragrant smoke that is believed to have a number of therapeutic benefits.

Types of Moxa Cones

There are several different types of moxa cones, each of which is believed to have its own unique benefits and uses.

Pure Moxa Cones

Pure moxa cones are made from 100% pure dried mugwort. These cones are believed to be the most potent form of moxa and are often used to treat chronic conditions, such as arthritis and musculoskeletal pain.

Smokeless Moxa Cones

Smokeless moxa cones are a newer form of moxa that is designed to reduce the amount of smoke produced during moxibustion. These cones are made from a mixture of dried mugwort and other herbs, such as sage or lavender. The addition of these herbs is believed to reduce the amount of smoke produced while still maintaining the therapeutic benefits of moxibustion.

Charcoal Moxa Cones

Charcoal moxa cones are made by adding a small amount of charcoal powder to the dried mugwort mixture. The charcoal is believed to enhance the therapeutic effects of moxibustion by increasing the heat and reducing the amount of smoke produced.

Wormwood and Mugwort Moxa Cones

Wormwood and mugwort moxa cones are made by combining dried wormwood and mugwort. Wormwood is believed to have additional therapeutic benefits, including the ability to kill parasites and promote digestion.

How Moxa Cones are Used in Moxibustion

Moxa cones are typically used in indirect moxibustion, which involves using a barrier, such as ginger or salt, to prevent the moxa from coming into direct contact with the skin. In indirect moxibustion, the moxa cone is placed on top of the barrier and allowed to burn until it is extinguished or until the patient experiences a strong sensation of warmth.

Moxa cones can also be used in direct moxibustion, which involves placing a small amount of moxa directly on the skin and lighting it. However, direct moxibustion with moxa cones is less common than indirect moxibustion.

Benefits of Moxa Cones

Moxa cones are believed to have a number of therapeutic benefits, including the ability to promote healing, alleviate pain, and stimulate the immune system. Moxa cones are often used to treat conditions such as arthritis, musculoskeletal pain, digestive disorders, and gynecological issues.

Moxa cones are also believed to promote relaxation and reduce stress. The fragrant smoke produced by burning moxa cones is believed to have a calming effect on the body and mind.

Moxa Boxes and Rollers

Moxibustion is a traditional Chinese medicine practice that involves the burning of dried mugwort on or near specific points on the body. In addition to moxa sticks and cones, there are other tools used in moxibustion, such as moxa boxes and rollers.

Moxa Boxes

Moxa boxes, also known as moxa cages or moxa cages with needles, are used in direct moxibustion. They are typically made from metal or bamboo and are designed to hold a small amount of moxa. The box is placed on the skin, and the moxa is lit. The heat from the burning moxa is then transmitted through the box and into the acupuncture point.

Moxa boxes are often used in combination with acupuncture needles. The needles are inserted into the acupuncture point, and the moxa box is placed on top of the needle. The heat from the burning moxa is then transmitted through the needle and into the acupuncture point.

Moxa boxes are believed to have a number of therapeutic benefits, including the ability to promote healing, alleviate pain, and stimulate the immune system. They are often used to treat conditions such as arthritis, musculoskeletal pain, digestive disorders, and gynecological issues.

Moxa Rollers

Moxa rollers are used in indirect moxibustion. They are typically made from metal or bamboo and are designed to hold a small amount of moxa. The roller is placed on the skin, and the moxa is lit. The roller is then moved back and forth along the skin, allowing the heat from the burning moxa to be transmitted through the roller and into the acupuncture point.

Moxa rollers are often used in combination with acupuncture needles or in areas where it is difficult to use moxa sticks or cones. They are believed to have similar therapeutic benefits to other forms of moxibustion, including the ability to promote healing, alleviate pain, and stimulate the immune system.

Safety Considerations for Moxa Boxes and Rollers

As with all forms of moxibustion, it is important to use caution when using moxa boxes and rollers. Burns can occur if the moxa is not applied properly, or if the heat is too intense. It is important to use a barrier, such as ginger or salt, to prevent the moxa from coming into direct contact with the skin.

It is also important to use high-quality moxa and to ensure that the moxa is stored in a dry, cool place. Moist or moldy moxa should never be used, as it can cause irritation or infection.

Essential Oils and Herbs

Moxibustion is a traditional Chinese medicine practice that involves the burning of dried mugwort on or near specific points on the body. In addition to the use of moxa sticks, cones, boxes, and rollers, essential oils and herbs can be used in conjunction with moxibustion to enhance its therapeutic effects.

Essential Oils

Essential oils are concentrated plant extracts that are often used in aromatherapy and other natural healing practices. When used in conjunction with moxibustion, essential oils can enhance the therapeutic effects of the treatment.

There are several essential oils that are commonly used in conjunction with moxibustion. These include:

Lavender Essential Oil

Lavender essential oil is often used to promote relaxation and reduce stress. When used in conjunction with moxibustion, lavender oil can enhance the calming effects of the treatment.

Peppermint Essential Oil

Peppermint essential oil is often used to promote digestion and alleviate nausea. When used in conjunction with moxibustion, peppermint oil can enhance the digestive benefits of the treatment.

Eucalyptus Essential Oil

Eucalyptus essential oil is often used to promote respiratory health and alleviate congestion. When used in conjunction with moxibustion, eucalyptus oil can enhance the respiratory benefits of the treatment.

Tea Tree Essential Oil

Tea tree essential oil is often used to promote skin health and alleviate inflammation. When used in conjunction with moxibustion, tea tree oil can enhance the skin benefits of the treatment.

Herbs

In addition to essential oils, herbs can also be used in conjunction with moxibustion. When used in conjunction with moxibustion, herbs can enhance the therapeutic effects of the treatment.

There are several herbs that are commonly used in conjunction with moxibustion. These include:

Ginger

Ginger is often used to promote digestion and alleviate nausea. When used in conjunction with moxibustion, ginger can enhance the digestive benefits of the treatment.

Cinnamon

Cinnamon is often used to promote circulation and alleviate pain. When used in conjunction with moxibustion, cinnamon can enhance the circulatory benefits of the treatment.

Angelica

Angelica is often used to promote women's health and alleviate menstrual pain. When used in conjunction with moxibustion, angelica can enhance the gynecological benefits of the treatment.

Licorice

Licorice is often used to promote respiratory health and alleviate inflammation. When used in conjunction with moxibustion, licorice can enhance the respiratory benefits of the treatment.

Safety Considerations for Essential Oils and Herbs

As with all forms of natural healing practices, it is important to use caution when using essential oils and herbs in conjunction with moxibustion. Some essential oils and herbs may interact with medications or may not be appropriate for certain individuals.

It is also important to use high-quality essential oils and herbs and to follow the instructions of a qualified practitioner. Essential oils and herbs should never be used in place of conventional medical treatments, and individuals should always consult with their healthcare provider before beginning any new natural healing practice.

Chapter Three

Preparing for Moxibustion

Moxibustion is a traditional Chinese medicine practice that involves the burning of dried mugwort on or near specific points on the body. It is believed to have a number of therapeutic benefits, including the ability to promote healing, alleviate pain, and stimulate the immune system. However, before undergoing moxibustion, it is important to properly prepare in order to ensure the best possible outcome.

Consult with a Qualified Practitioner

Before undergoing moxibustion, it is important to consult with a qualified practitioner. A qualified practitioner will be able to determine if moxibustion is appropriate for your condition and will be able to create a treatment plan tailored to your individual needs.

In addition, a qualified practitioner will be able to provide guidance on proper preparation for moxibustion. This may include dietary changes, lifestyle modifications, and other recommendations.

Wear Loose, Comfortable Clothing

When preparing for moxibustion, it is important to wear loose, comfortable clothing. This will allow the practitioner to access the areas of the body that need to be treated without restrictions.

It is also recommended to avoid wearing jewelry or other accessories that may interfere with the treatment.

Eat a Light Meal

Before undergoing moxibustion, it is recommended to eat a light meal. This will provide the body with the energy it needs for the treatment, while also preventing discomfort or nausea.

It is also important to avoid eating a heavy meal or consuming alcohol or caffeine prior to moxibustion, as these can interfere with the treatment.

Prepare the Treatment Area

When preparing for moxibustion, it is important to prepare the treatment area. This may include cleaning the skin with alcohol or another disinfectant, as well as applying a barrier, such as ginger or salt, to prevent the moxa from coming into direct contact with the skin.

It is also recommended to have a blanket or other cover nearby, as moxibustion can produce a strong sensation of warmth.

Relax and Breathe Deeply

During moxibustion, it is important to relax and breathe deeply. This will help to enhance the therapeutic effects of the treatment and promote a sense of calm and well-being.

In addition, it is important to communicate with the practitioner if you experience any discomfort or if the treatment becomes too intense.

Aftercare

After undergoing moxibustion, it is important to follow the aftercare instructions provided by the practitioner. This may include resting, drinking plenty of water, and avoiding strenuous activity for a period of time.

In addition, it is important to avoid exposure to extreme temperatures, such as hot showers or cold weather, as well as to avoid alcohol and caffeine for a period of time.

Creating a Safe and Comfortable Environment

Moxibustion is a traditional Chinese medicine practice that involves the burning of dried mugwort on or near specific points on the body. In order to create a safe and comfortable environment for moxibustion, there are several factors that should be taken into consideration.

Cleanliness and Sanitation

One of the most important factors in creating a safe and comfortable environment for moxibustion is cleanliness and sanitation. The treatment area should be clean and free from debris, and all equipment should be sanitized before and after each use.

It is also important to use high-quality moxa and to ensure that it is stored in a dry, cool place. Moist or moldy moxa should never be used, as it can cause irritation or infection.

Comfortable Temperature and Lighting

The treatment room should be kept at a comfortable temperature and lighting level. The room should be warm enough to prevent the patient from feeling cold during the treatment, but not so warm as to cause discomfort.

In addition, the lighting should be sufficient for the practitioner to see the treatment area and for the patient to feel comfortable and relaxed.

Comfortable Seating or Lying Surface

The patient should be provided with a comfortable seating or lying surface for the treatment. This may include a massage table, a recliner, or a bed, depending on the specific needs of the patient.

The seating or lying surface should be properly padded and should provide adequate support for the patient. The patient should also be provided with pillows or bolsters as needed for comfort.

Privacy and Confidentiality

Privacy and confidentiality are important factors in creating a safe and comfortable environment for moxibustion. The treatment room should be private and free from distractions, and the patient should be provided with a gown or other covering to ensure privacy during the treatment.

It is also important to maintain confidentiality regarding the patient's health information and treatment plan. This includes ensuring that all patient records are kept confidential and that patient information is not shared with unauthorized individuals.

Clear Communication

Clear communication between the practitioner and the patient is essential for creating a safe and comfortable environment for moxibustion. The practitioner should explain the treatment plan and any potential risks or side effects, and the patient should be encouraged to ask questions and express any concerns.

The practitioner should also be attentive to the patient's needs during the treatment, and should adjust the treatment as necessary to ensure the patient's comfort and safety.

Preparing the Patient

Moxibustion is a traditional Chinese medicine practice that involves the burning of dried mugwort on or near specific points on the body. Proper preparation of the patient is essential for a successful moxibustion treatment. By preparing the patient before the treatment, practitioners can ensure that the patient is comfortable and relaxed, which can enhance the therapeutic effects of the treatment.

Assessment of Medical History and Symptoms

Before beginning a moxibustion treatment, practitioners should assess the patient's medical history and symptoms. This may include a physical examination, as well as a review of the patient's medical records and any relevant diagnostic tests.

In addition, the practitioner should ask the patient about any symptoms they are experiencing, such as pain, fatigue, or anxiety. This information can help the practitioner to determine the appropriate moxibustion points and treatment plan.

Explain the Treatment

Before beginning the treatment, the practitioner should explain the moxibustion treatment to the patient. This may include a description of the procedure, the expected sensations, and any potential side effects or risks.

The practitioner should also answer any questions the patient may have, and should ensure that the patient is comfortable with the treatment plan before proceeding.

Prepare the Treatment Area

Before the treatment begins, the practitioner should prepare the treatment area. This may include cleaning the skin with alcohol or another disinfectant, as well as applying a barrier, such as ginger or salt, to prevent the moxa from coming into direct contact with the skin.

It is also recommended to have a blanket or other cover nearby, as moxibustion can produce a strong sensation of warmth.

Relaxation Techniques

Moxibustion can be a relaxing and therapeutic experience, but some patients may feel anxious or nervous before the treatment. Practitioners may use relaxation techniques, such as deep breathing or guided imagery, to help the patient feel more comfortable and relaxed before the treatment.

These techniques can also help to enhance the therapeutic effects of the treatment, as relaxation can promote a sense of calm and well-being.

Positioning the Patient

The positioning of the patient is an important factor in preparing for moxibustion. The patient should be positioned in a comfortable and relaxed position, such as lying down or sitting in a recliner.

The positioning should allow for easy access to the treatment area, and the patient should be provided with pillows or bolsters as needed for comfort.

Aftercare Instructions

After the moxibustion treatment is complete, the practitioner should provide the patient with aftercare instructions. This may include resting, drinking plenty of water, and avoiding strenuous activity for a period of time.

It is also important to avoid exposure to extreme temperatures, such as hot showers or cold weather, as well as to avoid alcohol and caffeine for a period of time.

Identifying Key Acupoints

Moxibustion is a traditional Chinese medicine practice that involves the burning of dried mugwort on or near specific points on the body. These points, known as acupoints, are believed to be located along pathways of energy, or meridians, that flow through the body. Identifying key acupoints is essential for a successful moxibustion treatment.

Traditional Chinese Medicine (TCM) Diagnosis

Before identifying key acupoints for moxibustion, a TCM diagnosis must be made. This involves assessing the patient's symptoms, medical history, and overall health to determine the underlying imbalances or disharmonies that are causing the symptoms.

Based on the TCM diagnosis, the practitioner can identify the meridians and acupoints that are most appropriate for treatment.

Meridian Theory

Meridian theory is a central concept in TCM, and it is used to identify key acupoints for moxibustion. The meridians are channels of energy that flow through the body, and they are associated with specific organs and bodily functions.

There are 12 main meridians, each associated with a different organ system, as well as eight extra meridians. Each meridian has specific acupoints that can be stimulated to promote healing and balance.

In addition to the meridians, there are also microsystems, such as the ear or hand, that are used for moxibustion treatments.

Palpation Techniques

Palpation techniques are often used to identify key acupoints for moxibustion. This involves using the fingers or hands to feel for areas of tenderness or tightness along the meridians.

These areas of tenderness or tightness, known as "ashi" points, are often indicative of blockages or imbalances in the flow of energy along the meridian. Stimulating these points with moxibustion can help to promote the flow of energy and alleviate symptoms.

Patient Feedback

Patient feedback is an important factor in identifying key acupoints for moxibustion. During the treatment, the patient may provide feedback about areas of discomfort or pain, or about areas that feel particularly sensitive or responsive to the moxibustion.

This feedback can help the practitioner to identify key acupoints and to adjust the treatment as needed to ensure the best possible outcome.

Combination of Techniques

In many cases, identifying key acupoints for moxibustion involves a combination of techniques. This may include palpation, patient feedback, and traditional meridian theory.

The practitioner may also use their intuition and clinical experience to identify key acupoints based on the individual needs of the patient.

Chapter Four

Moxibustion Techniques

Moxibustion is a traditional Chinese medicine practice that involves the burning of dried mugwort on or near specific points on the body. There are several different techniques for moxibustion, each with their own unique benefits and applications.

Direct Moxibustion

Direct moxibustion involves placing a small cone or ball of moxa directly on the skin at the acupuncture point. The moxa is then lit and allowed to burn until it is extinguished or until the patient feels a strong sensation of warmth.

Direct moxibustion is often used for localized conditions, such as joint pain or muscle stiffness, and can be particularly effective when combined with acupuncture.

Indirect Moxibustion

Indirect moxibustion involves placing a small amount of moxa on the acupuncture point and then using a barrier, such as ginger or salt, to prevent the moxa from coming into direct contact with the skin.

Indirect moxibustion can be performed using a variety of techniques, including a moxa stick, a moxa box or roller, or a moxa patch. This technique is often used for general tonification or for more systemic conditions, such as digestive disorders or respiratory problems.

Moxa Stick

A moxa stick, also known as a cigar, is a long, cylindrical piece of compressed moxa that can be lit and held close to the skin or waved over the acupuncture point. The heat from the moxa stick is transferred to the skin, producing a warming sensation that can promote circulation and relieve pain.

Moxa Box or Roller

A moxa box or roller is a small box or tube that contains burning moxa. The box or roller is placed on the acupuncture point and allowed to burn until it is extinguished or until the patient feels a strong sensation of warmth.

Moxa Patch

A moxa patch is a small adhesive pad that contains moxa. The patch is placed on the acupuncture point and allowed to heat up, producing a gentle warming sensation. Moxa patches are particularly useful for treating children or patients who are sensitive to heat or smoke.

Warm Needles

Warm needles involve heating the acupuncture needle with a small piece of moxa before inserting it into the acupuncture point. This can enhance the therapeutic effects of the acupuncture treatment by promoting circulation and reducing pain and inflammation.

Salt Moxibustion

Salt moxibustion involves placing a small amount of salt on the acupuncture point and then using moxa to heat the salt. This can help to enhance the therapeutic effects of the moxibustion treatment, particularly for patients with digestive disorders or other systemic conditions.

Direct Moxibustion

Direct moxibustion is a traditional Chinese medicine practice that involves placing a small cone or ball of moxa directly on the skin at the acupuncture point. The moxa is then lit and allowed to burn until it is extinguished or until the patient feels a strong sensation of warmth. Direct moxibustion is often used for localized conditions, such as joint pain or muscle stiffness, and can be particularly effective when combined with acupuncture.

Types of Direct Moxibustion

1. There are two main types of direct moxibustion: scarring and non-scarring. Scarring moxibustion involves burning the moxa until it creates a blister or small burn on the skin, which will then scar over and eventually heal. Non-scarring moxibustion, on the other hand, involves burning the moxa until it produces a strong sensation of warmth, but without causing any lasting damage to the skin.

Scarring Moxibustion

Scarring moxibustion is often used for chronic or stubborn conditions, such as arthritis or chronic pain. The scarring process can help to promote long-term healing by stimulating the body's natural healing processes and promoting the flow of energy through the affected area.

To perform scarring moxibustion, the practitioner will typically use a small cone or ball of moxa that is roughly the size of a grain of rice. The moxa is placed directly on the skin at the acupuncture point and lit, and allowed to burn until it creates a small blister or burn. The practitioner will then remove the moxa and treat the area with an antiseptic ointment to prevent infection.

Non-Scarring Moxibustion

Non-scarring moxibustion is often used for acute or mild conditions, such as a cold or flu. Non-scarring moxibustion can also be used for patients who are sensitive to heat or who may not be able to tolerate scarring moxibustion.

To perform non-scarring moxibustion, the practitioner will typically use a small cone or ball of moxa that is roughly the size of a grain of rice. The moxa is placed directly on the skin at the acupuncture point and lit, and allowed to burn until the patient feels a strong sensation of warmth. The practitioner will then remove the moxa and treat the area with an antiseptic ointment to prevent infection.

Benefits of Direct Moxibustion

Direct moxibustion can be particularly effective for localized conditions, such as joint pain or muscle stiffness. By applying heat directly to the affected area, direct moxibustion can help to promote circulation, reduce inflammation, and relieve pain.

In addition, direct moxibustion can be particularly effective when combined with acupuncture. By stimulating the acupuncture point with both moxibustion and acupuncture needles, the practitioner can enhance the therapeutic effects of the treatment and promote healing and balance throughout the body.

Potential Risks of Direct Moxibustion

As with any medical treatment, there are potential risks associated with direct moxibustion. The burning moxa can produce smoke and ash, which can be irritating to the eyes and lungs. Patients who have respiratory conditions or who are sensitive to smoke may not be good candidates for direct moxibustion.

In addition, scarring moxibustion can cause permanent scarring or discoloration of the skin. Patients who are concerned about scarring should discuss their options with their practitioner before undergoing direct moxibustion.

Indirect Moxibustion

Indirect moxibustion is a traditional Chinese medicine practice that involves placing a small amount of moxa on the acupuncture point and then using a barrier, such as ginger or salt, to prevent the moxa from coming into direct contact with the skin. Indirect moxibustion can be performed using a variety of techniques, including a moxa stick, a moxa box or roller, or a moxa patch. This technique is often used for general tonification or for more systemic conditions, such as digestive disorders or respiratory problems.

Types of Indirect Moxibustion

There are several different types of indirect moxibustion, each with its own unique benefits and applications.

Moxa Stick

A moxa stick, also known as a cigar, is a long, cylindrical piece of compressed moxa that can be lit and held close to the skin or waved over the acupuncture point. The heat from the moxa stick is transferred to the skin, producing a warming sensation that can promote circulation and relieve pain.

Moxa Box or Roller

A moxa box or roller is a small box or tube that contains burning moxa. The box or roller is placed on the acupuncture point and allowed to burn until it is extinguished or until the patient feels a strong sensation of warmth. Moxa boxes or rollers can be particularly effective for treating larger areas of the body, such as the back or abdomen.

Moxa Patch

A moxa patch is a small adhesive pad that contains moxa. The patch is placed on the acupuncture point and allowed to heat up, producing a gentle warming sensation. Moxa patches are particularly useful for treating children or patients who are sensitive to heat or smoke.

Ginger Moxibustion

Ginger moxibustion involves placing a slice of fresh ginger on the acupuncture point and then using moxa to heat the ginger. The ginger helps to direct the heat from the moxa to the acupuncture point, enhancing the therapeutic effects of the treatment.

Salt Moxibustion

Salt moxibustion involves placing a small amount of salt on the acupuncture point and then using moxa to heat the salt. This can help to enhance the therapeutic effects of the moxibustion treatment, particularly for patients with digestive disorders or other systemic conditions.

Benefits of Indirect Moxibustion

Indirect moxibustion can be particularly effective for general tonification or for more systemic conditions, such as digestive disorders or respiratory problems. By applying heat to the acupuncture point, indirect moxibustion can help to promote circulation, improve immune function, and relieve pain and inflammation.

Indirect moxibustion can also be a good option for patients who are sensitive to heat or smoke, or who may not be able to tolerate direct moxibustion. The use of barriers, such as ginger or salt, can help to prevent the moxa from coming into direct contact with the skin, making the treatment more comfortable for the patient.

Potential Risks of Indirect Moxibustion

As with any medical treatment, there are potential risks associated with indirect moxibustion. Patients who have respiratory conditions or who are sensitive to smoke may not be good candidates for indirect moxibustion.

In addition, indirect moxibustion can cause burns or skin irritation if the moxa is left on the skin for too long. Patients who experience any discomfort or irritation during the treatment should inform their practitioner immediately.

Needle Moxibustion

Needle moxibustion is a traditional Chinese medicine practice that involves using a small amount of moxa on the acupuncture needle to enhance the therapeutic effects of the treatment. Needle moxibustion is often used for chronic or stubborn conditions, such as chronic pain or infertility, and can be particularly effective when combined with acupuncture.

Types of Needle Moxibustion

1. There are two main types of needle moxibustion: direct and indirect. Direct needle moxibustion involves placing a small amount of moxa directly on the acupuncture needle, while indirect needle moxibustion involves using a moxa stick or box to heat the needle from a distance.

Direct Needle Moxibustion

Direct needle moxibustion is often used for chronic or stubborn conditions, such as chronic pain or infertility. To perform direct needle moxibustion, the practitioner will insert the acupuncture needle into the acupuncture point and then place a small amount of moxa on the needle. The moxa is then lit and allowed to burn until it is extinguished or until the patient feels a strong sensation of warmth.

Indirect Needle Moxibustion

Indirect needle moxibustion is often used for acute or mild conditions, such as a cold or flu. To perform indirect needle moxibustion, the practitioner will insert the acupuncture needle into the acupuncture point and then use a moxa stick or box to heat the needle from a distance. The heat from the moxa is transferred to the needle, producing a gentle warming sensation.

Benefits of Needle Moxibustion

Needle moxibustion can be particularly effective for chronic or stubborn conditions, such as chronic pain or infertility. By applying heat directly to the acupuncture point, needle moxibustion can help to promote circulation, reduce inflammation, and relieve pain.

In addition, needle moxibustion can be particularly effective when combined with acupuncture. By stimulating the acupuncture point with both moxibustion and acupuncture needles, the practitioner can enhance the therapeutic effects of the treatment and promote healing and balance throughout the body.

Potential Risks of Needle Moxibustion

As with any medical treatment, there are potential risks associated with needle moxibustion. Patients who have respiratory conditions or who are sensitive to smoke may not be good candidates for direct needle moxibustion.

In addition, needle moxibustion can cause burns or skin irritation if the moxa is left on the skin for too long. Patients who experience any discomfort or irritation during the treatment should inform their practitioner immediately.

Scarring and Non-Scarring Moxibustion

Scarring and non-scarring moxibustion are two different techniques used in traditional Chinese medicine. Both techniques involve the use of moxa, a dried herb that is burned near or on the skin to produce heat and stimulate specific acupuncture points. However, there are some key differences between the two techniques, particularly when it comes to the level of heat and the potential for scarring.

Scarring Moxibustion

Scarring moxibustion, also known as fire needle moxibustion, involves placing a small amount of moxa directly on the skin and burning it until it leaves a small, circular scar. The scarring is caused by the heat from the moxa, which burns the skin and creates a small wound. The wound then heals over time, leaving a scar that is believed to enhance the therapeutic effects of the treatment.

Scarring moxibustion is often used for chronic or stubborn conditions, such as arthritis or back pain. The scars are believed to enhance the therapeutic effects of the treatment by creating a permanent stimulation of the acupuncture point, which can help to promote circulation and relieve pain.

Non-Scarring Moxibustion

Non-scarring moxibustion, also known as indirect moxibustion, involves using a barrier, such as ginger or salt, to prevent the moxa from coming into direct contact with the skin. The moxa is burned near the skin, producing a gentle warming sensation that can promote circulation and relieve pain.

Non-scarring moxibustion is often used for general tonification or for more systemic conditions, such as digestive disorders or respiratory problems. By applying heat to the acupuncture point, non-scarring moxibustion can help to promote circulation, improve immune function, and relieve pain and inflammation.

Benefits and Risks of Scarring Moxibustion

Scarring moxibustion can be particularly effective for chronic or stubborn conditions, such as arthritis or back pain. The scars created by the treatment are believed to enhance the therapeutic effects of the treatment by creating a permanent stimulation of the acupuncture point.

However, scarring moxibustion does carry some potential risks. Patients who are prone to scarring or who have sensitive skin may not be good candidates for this technique. In addition, there is a risk of infection if the wound is not properly cared for after the treatment.

Benefits and Risks of Non-Scarring Moxibustion

Non-scarring moxibustion can be a good option for patients who are sensitive to heat or smoke, or who may not be able to tolerate direct moxibustion. The use of barriers, such as ginger or salt, can help to prevent the moxa from coming into direct contact with the skin, making the treatment more comfortable for the patient.

Non-scarring moxibustion is generally considered to be safe, although there is a risk of burns or skin irritation if the moxa is left on the skin for too long. Patients who experience any discomfort or irritation during the treatment should inform their practitioner immediately.

Chapter Five

Conditions and Diseases Treated by Moxibustion

Moxibustion is a traditional Chinese medicine practice that involves burning a dried herb called moxa near or on the skin to stimulate specific acupuncture points. Moxibustion has been used for centuries to treat a variety of conditions and diseases, and is often used in combination with other therapies, such as acupuncture.

Here are some of the conditions and diseases that can be treated with moxibustion:

Pain

Moxibustion can be used to treat a variety of pain conditions, including chronic back pain, arthritis, and menstrual cramps. By stimulating the acupuncture points, moxibustion can help to promote circulation, reduce inflammation, and relieve pain.

Digestive Disorders

Moxibustion can be used to treat a variety of digestive disorders, including irritable bowel syndrome (IBS) and acid reflux. By stimulating the acupuncture points, moxibustion can help to improve digestion, reduce inflammation, and relieve pain and discomfort.

Respiratory Disorders

Moxibustion can be used to treat a variety of respiratory disorders, including asthma, bronchitis, and chronic obstructive pulmonary disease (COPD). By stimulating the acupuncture points, moxibustion can help to improve lung function, reduce inflammation, and relieve coughing and wheezing.

Infertility

Moxibustion can be used to treat infertility in both men and women. By stimulating the acupuncture points, moxibustion can help to improve blood flow to the reproductive organs, regulate hormone levels, and improve the quality of sperm and eggs.

Stress and Anxiety

Moxibustion can be used to treat stress and anxiety by promoting relaxation and reducing tension in the body. By stimulating the acupuncture points, moxibustion can help to regulate the nervous system and promote a sense of calm and wellbeing.

Skin Disorders

Moxibustion can be used to treat a variety of skin disorders, including eczema, psoriasis, and acne. By stimulating the acupuncture points, moxibustion can help to reduce inflammation, improve circulation, and promote healing and regeneration of the skin.

Menopause Symptoms

Moxibustion can be used to treat symptoms of menopause, including hot flashes, night sweats, and mood swings. By stimulating the acupuncture points, moxibustion can help to regulate hormone levels and reduce the severity and frequency of menopausal symptoms.

Pain Relief and Management

Pain is a common condition that affects millions of people worldwide. Pain can be acute, such as the pain from a sprained ankle, or chronic, such as the pain from arthritis. While there are many treatments available for pain relief, some patients may choose to explore alternative therapies, such as moxibustion.

Moxibustion is a traditional Chinese medicine practice that involves burning a dried herb called moxa near or on the skin to stimulate specific acupuncture points. Moxibustion has been used for centuries to treat pain, and is often used in combination with other therapies, such as acupuncture.

Here are some ways in which moxibustion can be used for pain relief and management:

Back Pain

Moxibustion can be used to treat chronic back pain, a common condition that affects millions of people worldwide. By stimulating the acupuncture points, moxibustion can help to improve circulation, reduce inflammation, and relieve pain.

Arthritis

Moxibustion can be used to treat arthritis, a chronic condition that affects the joints and causes pain and inflammation. By stimulating the acupuncture points, moxibustion can help to reduce inflammation, improve circulation, and relieve pain.

Headaches

Moxibustion can be used to treat headaches, a common condition that affects millions of people worldwide. By stimulating the acupuncture points, moxibustion can help to reduce tension and promote relaxation, which can help to relieve headaches.

Menstrual Cramps

Moxibustion can be used to treat menstrual cramps, a common condition that affects many women. By stimulating the acupuncture points, moxibustion can help to improve circulation and relieve pain and discomfort associated with menstrual cramps.

Sports Injuries

Moxibustion can be used to treat sports injuries, such as sprains and strains. By stimulating the acupuncture points, moxibustion can help to improve circulation, reduce inflammation, and promote healing and recovery.

Neuropathic Pain

Moxibustion can be used to treat neuropathic pain, a chronic condition that affects the nerves and causes pain and discomfort. By stimulating the acupuncture points, moxibustion can help to regulate the nervous system and reduce pain and discomfort associated with neuropathic pain.

Fibromyalgia

Moxibustion can be used to treat fibromyalgia, a chronic condition that causes widespread pain and fatigue. By stimulating the acupuncture points, moxibustion can help to reduce pain and fatigue associated with fibromyalgia, and promote relaxation and wellbeing.

Digestive Disorders

Digestive disorders are a common health concern that can have a significant impact on an individual's quality of life. These disorders can range from mild discomfort to more serious conditions that require medical attention. Traditional Chinese medicine (TCM) offers various treatment options for digestive disorders, including moxibustion.

Moxibustion is a traditional Chinese medicine practice that involves burning a dried herb called moxa near or on the skin to stimulate specific acupuncture points. Moxibustion has been used for centuries to treat a variety of conditions, including digestive disorders. Here are some ways in which moxibustion can be used for digestive disorders:

Irritable Bowel Syndrome (IBS)

Moxibustion can be used to treat IBS, a common digestive disorder that affects the large intestine. By stimulating the acupuncture points, moxibustion can help to improve digestion, reduce inflammation, and relieve pain and discomfort associated with IBS.

Acid Reflux

Moxibustion can be used to treat acid reflux, a digestive disorder that causes heartburn and acid regurgitation. By stimulating the acupuncture points, moxibustion can help to improve digestion, reduce inflammation, and relieve symptoms associated with acid reflux.

Crohn's Disease

Moxibustion can be used to treat Crohn's disease, a chronic inflammatory bowel disease that affects the digestive tract. By stimulating the acupuncture points, moxibustion can help to reduce inflammation, improve digestion, and relieve symptoms associated with Crohn's disease.

Ulcerative Colitis

Moxibustion can be used to treat ulcerative colitis, a chronic inflammatory bowel disease that affects the colon and rectum. By stimulating the acupuncture points, moxibustion can help to reduce inflammation, improve digestion, and relieve symptoms associated with ulcerative colitis.

Constipation

Moxibustion can be used to treat constipation, a common digestive disorder that affects many people. By stimulating the acupuncture points, moxibustion can help to improve digestion, promote bowel movements, and relieve symptoms associated with constipation.

Diarrhea

Moxibustion can be used to treat diarrhea, a common digestive disorder that can be caused by a variety of factors. By stimulating the acupuncture points, moxibustion can help to improve digestion, reduce inflammation, and relieve symptoms associated with diarrhea.

Indigestion

Moxibustion can be used to treat indigestion, a common digestive disorder that can be caused by a variety of factors. By stimulating the acupuncture points, moxibustion can help to improve digestion, reduce inflammation, and relieve symptoms associated with indigestion.

Respiratory Issues

Respiratory issues are a common concern that can range from mild discomfort to more serious conditions that require medical attention. Traditional Chinese medicine (TCM) offers various treatment options for respiratory issues, including moxibustion.

Moxibustion is a traditional Chinese medicine practice that involves burning a dried herb called moxa near or on the skin to stimulate specific acupuncture points. Moxibustion has been used for centuries to treat a variety of conditions, including respiratory issues. Here are some ways in which moxibustion can be used for respiratory issues:

Asthma

Moxibustion can be used to treat asthma, a common respiratory condition that affects the airways. By stimulating the acupuncture points, moxibustion can help to reduce inflammation, improve lung function, and relieve symptoms associated with asthma.

Bronchitis

Moxibustion can be used to treat bronchitis, a respiratory condition that causes inflammation of the bronchial tubes. By stimulating the acupuncture points, moxibustion can help to reduce inflammation, improve lung function, and relieve symptoms associated with bronchitis.

Sinusitis

Moxibustion can be used to treat sinusitis, a condition that causes inflammation of the sinuses. By stimulating the acupuncture points, moxibustion can help to reduce inflammation, improve sinus function, and relieve symptoms associated with sinusitis.

Chronic Obstructive Pulmonary Disease (COPD)

Moxibustion can be used to treat COPD, a chronic respiratory disease that affects the lungs. By stimulating the acupuncture points, moxibustion can help to improve lung function, reduce inflammation, and relieve symptoms associated with COPD.

Allergies

Moxibustion can be used to treat allergies, a common respiratory condition that can cause a variety of symptoms. By stimulating the acupuncture points, moxibustion can help to reduce inflammation, improve lung function, and relieve symptoms associated with allergies.

Common Cold and Flu

Moxibustion can be used to treat the common cold and flu, respiratory conditions that can cause a variety of symptoms. By stimulating the acupuncture points, moxibustion can help to reduce inflammation, improve lung function, and relieve symptoms associated with the common cold and flu.

Pneumonia

Moxibustion can be used to treat pneumonia, a respiratory condition that causes inflammation of the lungs. By stimulating the acupuncture points, moxibustion can help to reduce inflammation, improve lung function, and relieve symptoms associated with pneumonia.

Women's Health and Fertility

Women's health and fertility are important concerns that can have a significant impact on an individual's quality of life. Traditional Chinese medicine (TCM) offers various treatment options for women's health and fertility, including moxibustion.

Moxibustion is a traditional Chinese medicine practice that involves burning a dried herb called moxa near or on the skin to stimulate specific acupuncture points. Moxibustion has been used for centuries to treat a variety of conditions, including women's health and fertility. Here are some ways in which moxibustion can be used for women's health and fertility:

Menstrual Issues

Moxibustion can be used to treat menstrual issues, such as irregular periods, painful periods, and heavy bleeding. By stimulating the acupuncture points, moxibustion can help to regulate the menstrual cycle, improve blood circulation, and relieve symptoms associated with menstrual issues.

Menopause

Moxibustion can be used to treat menopause, a natural process that causes a decline in hormone levels in women. By stimulating the acupuncture points, moxibustion can help to regulate hormone levels, reduce hot flashes, and relieve symptoms associated with menopause.

Polycystic Ovary Syndrome (PCOS)

Moxibustion can be used to treat PCOS, a common hormonal disorder that affects women of reproductive age. By stimulating the acupuncture points, moxibustion can help to regulate hormone levels, improve ovarian function, and relieve symptoms associated with PCOS.

Endometriosis

Moxibustion can be used to treat endometriosis, a condition in which tissue similar to the lining of the uterus grows outside of the uterus. By stimulating the acupuncture points, moxibustion can help to reduce inflammation, improve blood circulation, and relieve symptoms associated with endometriosis.

Infertility

Moxibustion can be used to treat infertility, a condition in which a couple is unable to conceive after trying for a certain period of time. By stimulating the acupuncture points, moxibustion can help to regulate hormone levels, improve ovarian function, and increase the chances of conception.

Pregnancy and Labor

Moxibustion can be used during pregnancy to alleviate symptoms such as morning sickness, back pain, and fatigue. Moxibustion can also be used during labor to help stimulate contractions and relieve pain.

Postpartum Recovery

Moxibustion can be used postpartum to help the body recover from childbirth. By stimulating the acupuncture points, moxibustion can help to improve blood circulation, reduce inflammation, and promote healing.

Chapter Six

Combining Moxibustion with Other Therapies

Moxibustion is a traditional Chinese medicine practice that involves burning a dried herb called moxa near or on the skin to stimulate specific acupuncture points. Moxibustion has been used for centuries to treat a variety of conditions and is often combined with other therapies for maximum benefit.

Here are some therapies that can be combined with moxibustion:

Acupuncture

Acupuncture is another traditional Chinese medicine practice that involves inserting needles into specific acupuncture points to promote healing and relieve pain. Acupuncture can be combined with moxibustion to enhance the benefits of both therapies. Together, acupuncture and moxibustion can help to promote blood circulation, reduce inflammation, and relieve pain.

Massage

Massage therapy involves manipulating the soft tissues of the body to promote relaxation and reduce stress. Massage therapy can be combined with moxibustion to enhance the benefits of both therapies. Together, massage therapy and moxibustion can help to promote blood circulation, reduce tension in the muscles, and relieve pain.

Herbal Medicine

Herbal medicine involves using plant-based remedies to promote healing and relieve symptoms. Herbal medicine can be combined with moxibustion to enhance the benefits of both therapies. Together, herbal medicine and moxibustion can help to promote blood circulation, reduce inflammation, and relieve pain.

Cupping

Cupping is a therapy that involves placing cups on the skin to create a suction effect. Cupping can be combined with moxibustion to enhance the benefits of both therapies. Together, cupping and moxibustion can help to promote blood circulation, reduce inflammation, and relieve pain.

Dietary Therapy

Dietary therapy involves making dietary changes to promote health and well-being. Dietary therapy can be combined with moxibustion to enhance the benefits of both therapies. Together, dietary therapy and moxibustion can help to promote blood circulation, reduce inflammation, and relieve pain.

Acupuncture

Acupuncture is a traditional Chinese medicine practice that involves inserting thin needles into specific acupuncture points on the body to promote healing and relieve pain. Acupuncture has been used for centuries to treat a variety of conditions and is often combined with other therapies, such as moxibustion, for maximum benefit.

Acupuncture is based on the concept of qi (pronounced "chee"), which is the vital energy that flows through the body along pathways called meridians. According to traditional Chinese medicine, illness and pain occur when qi is blocked or out of balance. By stimulating specific acupuncture points, acupuncture can help to restore the flow of qi and promote healing.

Acupuncture needles are very thin, typically about the width of a human hair. They are inserted into specific acupuncture points, which are located along the meridians of the body. Acupuncture points are typically located on the skin, but they can also be located on the ears, scalp, and other parts of the body.

Acupuncture is generally considered safe when performed by a licensed and experienced practitioner. The needles are sterile and single-use, which helps to reduce the risk of infection. Some patients may experience mild side effects, such as soreness, bruising, or bleeding at the site of the needles, but these side effects are typically minor and resolve quickly.

Acupuncture can be used to treat a variety of conditions, including:

Pain

Acupuncture is often used to relieve pain, such as back pain, neck pain, and joint pain. By stimulating the acupuncture points, acupuncture can help to promote the release of endorphins, which are the body's natural painkillers.

Stress and Anxiety

Acupuncture can be used to reduce stress and anxiety. By stimulating the acupuncture points, acupuncture can help to promote relaxation and reduce tension in the muscles.

Digestive Issues

Acupuncture can be used to treat digestive issues, such as irritable bowel syndrome (IBS) and acid reflux. By stimulating the acupuncture points, acupuncture can help to regulate the digestive system and improve digestion.

Respiratory Issues

Acupuncture can be used to treat respiratory issues, such as asthma and allergies. By stimulating the acupuncture points, acupuncture can help to regulate the respiratory system and reduce inflammation in the airways.

Women's Health

Acupuncture can be used to treat women's health issues, such as menstrual issues, menopause, and infertility. By stimulating the acupuncture points, acupuncture can help to regulate hormone levels, improve ovarian function, and relieve symptoms associated with women's health issues.

Substance Abuse

Acupuncture can be used to treat substance abuse, such as addiction to drugs or alcohol. By stimulating the acupuncture points, acupuncture can help to reduce cravings and promote relaxation during the withdrawal process.

Massage and Cupping

Massage and cupping are two traditional healing therapies that have been used for centuries to promote healing and relieve pain. These therapies can be used in conjunction with moxibustion to enhance the overall healing experience.

Massage Therapy

Massage therapy involves manipulating the soft tissues of the body, such as muscles and tendons, to promote relaxation and reduce stress. Massage therapy has been shown to have numerous health benefits, including:

Reducing muscle tension and soreness

Improving circulation

Reducing stress and anxiety

Improving range of motion

Reducing pain

There are many different types of massage therapy, including Swedish massage, deep tissue massage, and sports massage. During a massage therapy session, the therapist will use a variety of techniques, including kneading, tapping, and friction, to manipulate the muscles and tissues of the body.

Cupping Therapy

Cupping therapy involves placing cups on the skin to create a suction effect. The cups can be made of glass, bamboo, or other materials. Cupping therapy has been shown to have numerous health benefits, including:

Increasing blood flow

Reducing inflammation

Relaxing muscles

Relieving pain

Boosting the immune system

1. There are two main types of cupping therapy: dry cupping and wet cupping. Dry cupping involves placing cups on the skin and creating a

suction effect without drawing blood. Wet cupping involves creating a small incision in the skin and then placing the cup on the skin to draw out a small amount of blood.

Moxibustion and Massage Therapy

Moxibustion and massage therapy can be combined to enhance the benefits of both therapies. Moxibustion can be used to promote blood circulation and reduce inflammation, while massage therapy can be used to manipulate the muscles and tissues of the body to reduce tension and promote relaxation.

During a moxibustion and massage therapy session, the therapist may use moxa sticks or cones to stimulate specific acupuncture points on the body. The therapist will then use massage techniques to manipulate the muscles and tissues of the body, promoting relaxation and reducing tension.

Moxibustion and Cupping Therapy

Moxibustion and cupping therapy can also be combined to enhance the benefits of both therapies. Moxibustion can be used to promote blood circulation and reduce inflammation, while cupping therapy can be used to create a suction effect on the skin, promoting blood flow and reducing inflammation.

During a moxibustion and cupping therapy session, the therapist may use moxa sticks or cones to stimulate specific acupuncture points on the body. The therapist will then place cups on the skin to create a suction effect, promoting blood flow and reducing inflammation.

Herbal Medicine

Herbal medicine is a traditional healing therapy that involves using plant-based materials to promote healing and relieve pain. Herbal medicine can be used in conjunction with moxibustion to enhance the overall healing experience.

Herbal medicine has been used for centuries to treat a variety of conditions, including:

Digestive issues

Respiratory issues

Women's health issues

Pain management

Immune system support

Herbal medicine involves using the whole plant or specific plant parts, such as leaves, stems, or roots, to create teas, tinctures, or supplements. Different plants have different medicinal properties, and each plant can be used to treat specific conditions.

During an herbal medicine and moxibustion session, the practitioner may use moxa sticks or cones to stimulate specific acupuncture points on the body. The practitioner will then recommend specific herbal remedies to the patient to promote healing and relieve pain.

There are many different types of herbal remedies that can be used in conjunction with moxibustion, including:

1. Ginger: Ginger is often used to treat digestive issues, such as nausea and bloating. It can also be used to relieve pain and reduce inflammation.

2. Echinacea: Echinacea is often used to boost the immune system and prevent infections.

3. Chamomile: Chamomile is often used to promote relaxation and reduce stress and anxiety.

4. Ginkgo biloba: Ginkgo biloba is often used to improve circulation and promote cognitive function.

5. St. John's Wort: St. John's Wort is often used to treat depression and anxiety.

Herbal remedies should be used under the guidance of a licensed and experienced practitioner to ensure safety and effectiveness. It is important to note that herbal remedies can interact with certain medications, so patients should always consult with their healthcare provider before using any herbal remedies.

Chapter Seven

Moxibustion for Prevention and Wellness

Moxibustion is a traditional healing therapy that involves burning dried mugwort on or near specific acupuncture points on the body. This therapy has been used for centuries to promote healing and relieve pain. While moxibustion is often used to treat specific conditions, it can also be used as a preventative measure to promote overall wellness.

Moxibustion for Prevention

Moxibustion can be used as a preventative measure to promote overall health and prevent illness. By stimulating specific acupuncture points on the body, moxibustion can promote blood circulation, boost the immune system, and balance the body's energy flow.

Studies have shown that regular moxibustion treatments can help prevent a variety of health conditions, including:

Respiratory infections

Digestive issues

Women's health issues

Musculoskeletal pain

Neurological conditions

Moxibustion for Wellness

Moxibustion can also be used to promote overall wellness and reduce stress. By stimulating specific acupuncture points on the body, moxibustion can promote relaxation and reduce tension.

Studies have shown that regular moxibustion treatments can help:

Reduce stress and anxiety

Promote relaxation

Improve sleep quality

Enhance overall well-being

During a moxibustion treatment for prevention or wellness, the practitioner may use moxa sticks or cones to stimulate specific acupuncture points on the body. The patient will typically lie down or sit comfortably during the treatment, and the practitioner will place the moxa on or near specific points on the body. The moxa will then be lit, and the patient will feel a warm, pleasant sensation as the moxa burns.

It is important to note that moxibustion should only be performed by licensed and experienced practitioners to ensure safety and effectiveness. Patients who are interested in using moxibustion for prevention or wellness should discuss their options with their practitioner and determine if this technique is right for their specific needs.

In addition to moxibustion, other preventative and wellness strategies can also be used to promote overall health, including:

Regular exercise

Healthy diet

Adequate sleep

Stress management techniques, such as meditation or yoga

Boosting Immune Function

The immune system plays a vital role in protecting the body from illness and disease. It is responsible for identifying and fighting off harmful viruses, bacteria, and other foreign invaders that can make us sick. Moxibustion is a traditional healing therapy that has been used for centuries to boost immune function and promote overall health.

Moxibustion and the Immune System

Moxibustion works by stimulating specific acupuncture points on the body using burning dried mugwort. When applied to specific acupuncture points, moxibustion can stimulate the immune system, promote blood circulation, and balance the body's energy flow. This stimulation can help boost immune function and improve overall health.

Studies have shown that moxibustion can help boost immune function in a variety of ways, including:

1. Increasing the production of immune cells: Moxibustion has been shown to increase the production of immune cells, such as white blood cells, which are responsible for fighting off infections and other foreign invaders.

2. Enhancing the immune response: Moxibustion has been shown to enhance the immune response by increasing the activity of immune cells and promoting the release of immune-boosting chemicals in the body.

3. Reducing inflammation: Moxibustion has been shown to reduce inflammation in the body, which can help improve immune function and reduce the risk of chronic disease.

Moxibustion and Immune Function

Moxibustion can be used to promote immune function and overall health in a variety of ways. Here are some of the ways that moxibustion can be used to boost immune function:

4. Prevention: Moxibustion can be used as a preventative measure to promote overall health and prevent illness. By stimulating specific acupuncture points on the body, moxibustion can promote blood circulation, boost the immune system, and balance the body's energy flow.

5. Treatment: Moxibustion can also be used to treat specific conditions that may be compromising immune function, such as chronic stress, anxiety, or chronic pain.

6. Maintenance: Regular moxibustion treatments can be used to maintain immune function and promote overall health. Studies have shown that regular moxibustion treatments can help prevent a variety of health conditions, including respiratory infections, digestive issues, and musculoskeletal pain.

It is important to note that moxibustion should only be performed by licensed and experienced practitioners to ensure safety and effectiveness. Patients who are interested in using moxibustion to boost immune function should discuss their options with their practitioner and determine if this technique is right for their specific needs.

In addition to moxibustion, other strategies can also be used to boost immune function and promote overall health, including:

Regular exercise

Healthy diet

Adequate sleep

Stress management techniques, such as meditation or yoga

Enhancing Energy Levels

Feeling sluggish and tired can be a frustrating experience that can impact our productivity, mood, and overall quality of life. While there are many strategies for enhancing energy levels, such as regular exercise, a healthy diet, and adequate sleep, moxibustion can also be used as a natural way to boost energy and promote overall vitality.

Moxibustion and Energy

Moxibustion is a traditional healing therapy that involves burning dried mugwort on specific acupuncture points on the body. When applied to these points, moxibustion can stimulate the flow of qi (energy) throughout the body and help restore balance to the body's energy flow. This stimulation can help enhance energy levels and promote overall vitality.

Studies have shown that moxibustion can help enhance energy levels in a variety of ways, including:

1. Stimulating the nervous system: Moxibustion can stimulate the nervous system and promote the release of energy-boosting chemicals in the body, such as endorphins.

2. Improving circulation: Moxibustion can improve blood circulation, which can help deliver more oxygen and nutrients to the body's cells, resulting in increased energy levels.

3. Boosting immunity: Moxibustion can help boost immune function, which can help protect the body from illness and disease, and promote overall vitality.

Moxibustion and Energy Levels

Moxibustion can be used to enhance energy levels in a variety of ways. Here are some of the ways that moxibustion can be used to boost energy levels:

4. Treatment: Moxibustion can be used to treat specific conditions that may be impacting energy levels, such as chronic fatigue, depression, or anxiety.

5. Prevention: Moxibustion can be used as a preventative measure to promote overall health and prevent conditions that may impact energy levels, such as stress or illness.

6. Maintenance: Regular moxibustion treatments can be used to maintain energy levels and promote overall vitality. Studies have shown that regular moxibustion treatments can help improve energy levels, reduce stress, and promote a sense of well-being.

It is important to note that moxibustion should only be performed by licensed and experienced practitioners to ensure safety and effectiveness. Patients who are interested in using moxibustion to enhance energy levels should discuss their options with their practitioner and determine if this technique is right for their specific needs.

In addition to moxibustion, other strategies can also be used to enhance energy levels and promote overall vitality, including:

7. Regular exercise: Exercise can help boost energy levels and promote overall health.

8. Healthy diet: Eating a balanced diet that is rich in nutrients can help enhance energy levels and promote overall vitality.

9. Adequate sleep: Getting enough sleep is essential for promoting energy levels and overall health.

10. Stress management techniques: Stress can impact energy levels, so incorporating stress management techniques, such as meditation or yoga, can help promote a sense of calm and boost energy levels.

Reducing Stress and Anxiety

Stress and anxiety are common experiences that can negatively impact our physical, emotional, and mental health. While there are many strategies for reducing stress and anxiety, including exercise, meditation, and therapy, moxibustion can also be used as a natural way to promote relaxation and reduce stress and anxiety.

Moxibustion and Stress

Moxibustion is a traditional healing therapy that involves burning dried mugwort on specific acupuncture points on the body. When applied to these points, moxibustion can stimulate the flow of qi (energy) throughout the body and help restore balance to the body's energy flow. This stimulation can help reduce stress and promote relaxation.

Studies have shown that moxibustion can help reduce stress and anxiety in a variety of ways, including:

1. Promoting relaxation: Moxibustion can help promote relaxation by stimulating the release of endorphins, which are natural painkillers and mood enhancers.

2. Reducing inflammation: Chronic inflammation can contribute to stress and anxiety, and moxibustion has been shown to reduce inflammation in the body.

3. Regulating the nervous system: Moxibustion can help regulate the nervous system, which can help reduce stress and anxiety.

Moxibustion and Anxiety

Moxibustion can be used to reduce anxiety in a variety of ways. Here are some of the ways that moxibustion can be used to promote relaxation and reduce anxiety:

4. Treatment: Moxibustion can be used to treat specific conditions that may be contributing to anxiety, such as depression or insomnia.

5. Prevention: Moxibustion can be used as a preventative measure to promote relaxation and prevent conditions that may contribute to anxiety, such as stress or illness.

6. Maintenance: Regular moxibustion treatments can be used to maintain relaxation and promote a sense of well-being. Studies have shown that regular moxibustion treatments can help reduce anxiety, improve sleep, and promote overall mental health.

It is important to note that moxibustion should only be performed by licensed and experienced practitioners to ensure safety and effectiveness. Patients who are interested in using moxibustion to reduce stress and anxiety should discuss their options with their practitioner and determine if this technique is right for their specific needs.

In addition to moxibustion, other strategies can also be used to reduce stress and anxiety, including:

7. Meditation and mindfulness: These practices can help promote relaxation and reduce stress and anxiety.

8. Exercise: Regular exercise can help reduce stress and promote overall well-being.

9. Therapy: Talk therapy can be used to explore and address the root causes of stress and anxiety.

10. Stress management techniques: Incorporating stress management techniques, such as deep breathing or progressive muscle relaxation, can help reduce stress and promote relaxation.

Chapter Eight

Moxibustion Safety and Precautions

Moxibustion is a traditional Chinese medicine technique that involves the burning of dried mugwort on specific acupuncture points on the body. While moxibustion can be a safe and effective treatment option, it is important to take certain safety precautions to ensure that the treatment is performed safely and effectively.

Here are some of the safety precautions that patients and practitioners should consider when performing moxibustion:

Seek Professional Care

Moxibustion should only be performed by a licensed and experienced practitioner. Patients should seek out a qualified practitioner who has experience in moxibustion and other traditional Chinese medicine techniques.

Check for Allergies

Before beginning moxibustion, patients should check for allergies to mugwort or other herbs that may be used in the treatment. If a patient has an allergy to mugwort, they may be at risk of an allergic reaction during the treatment.

Avoid Sensitive Areas

When performing moxibustion, practitioners should avoid sensitive areas of the body, such as the face, eyes, and genitals. Burning moxa in these areas can cause serious injury.

Monitor Temperature

During moxibustion, the temperature of the burning moxa should be monitored to prevent burns and other injuries. The practitioner should use a temperature monitor to ensure that the moxa is not too hot for the patient.

Use Clean Tools

Practitioners should use clean and sterile tools when performing moxibustion. This can help prevent infection and other complications.

Avoid Inflammation

Moxibustion should be avoided in areas of the body that are inflamed or infected. Burning moxa on these areas can worsen the inflammation and cause further damage.

Monitor Patient Reactions

During moxibustion, the practitioner should monitor the patient's reactions to the treatment. If the patient experiences pain, discomfort, or other adverse reactions, the treatment should be stopped immediately.

Pregnant Women

Moxibustion should be used with caution in pregnant women. While moxibustion can be a safe and effective treatment option for certain conditions during pregnancy, it is important to consult with a qualified practitioner and follow proper safety precautions.

Patient Health History

Patients should inform their practitioner of any health conditions, medications, or allergies they may have. This can help the practitioner determine if moxibustion is a safe and effective treatment option for the patient.

Avoid DIY Moxibustion

Patients should avoid performing moxibustion on themselves at home. Moxibustion should only be performed by a licensed and experienced practitioner.

Possible Side Effects and Risks

Moxibustion is a traditional Chinese medicine technique that involves the burning of dried mugwort on specific acupuncture points on the body. While moxibustion is generally considered safe when performed by a licensed and experienced practitioner, there are some possible side effects and risks to be aware of.

Here are some of the possible side effects and risks associated with moxibustion:

Burns and Skin Irritation

One of the most common risks associated with moxibustion is burns and skin irritation. The burning moxa can cause the skin to become red and irritated, and in some cases, it can cause burns. This risk can be minimized by using the proper techniques and tools, monitoring the temperature of the moxa, and avoiding sensitive areas of the body.

Smoke and Odor

Moxibustion produces smoke and a strong odor, which can be unpleasant for some patients. While this is generally not a serious risk, it can be a concern for patients with respiratory conditions or sensitivities.

Allergic Reactions

Some patients may be allergic to mugwort or other herbs that are used in moxibustion. This can cause symptoms such as itching, rash, and difficulty breathing. Patients should inform their practitioner of any allergies before beginning moxibustion.

Infection

If the tools used in moxibustion are not properly sterilized, there is a risk of infection. This can lead to skin infections or other complications.

Pregnancy

Moxibustion should be used with caution in pregnant women. While moxibustion can be a safe and effective treatment option for certain conditions during pregnancy, it is important to consult with a qualified practitioner and follow proper safety precautions.

Adverse Reactions

In rare cases, patients may experience adverse reactions to moxibustion, such as dizziness, nausea, or fainting. If a patient experiences these symptoms, the treatment should be stopped immediately.

Contraindications

Moxibustion should not be performed on areas of the body that are inflamed or infected. It should also be avoided in patients with certain medical conditions, such as high fever or acute illness. Patients with certain medical devices, such as pacemakers, should also avoid moxibustion.

While moxibustion can be a safe and effective treatment option, it is important for patients and practitioners to be aware of the possible side effects and risks. By following proper safety precautions and using the right techniques and tools, the risk of these side effects and risks can be minimized. Patients should also inform their practitioner of any health conditions, medications, or allergies they may have to ensure that moxibustion is a safe and effective treatment option for them.

Contraindications

Moxibustion is a traditional Chinese medicine technique that involves the burning of dried mugwort on specific acupuncture points on the body. While moxibustion can be a safe and effective treatment option for many conditions, there are some contraindications to be aware of. Contraindications are specific situations or conditions in which a treatment should not be used or should be used with caution.

Here are some of the contraindications associated with moxibustion:

Inflammation or Infection

Moxibustion should not be performed on areas of the body that are inflamed or infected. This can lead to further irritation or spread the infection.

Fever or Acute Illness

Moxibustion should not be performed on patients with a high fever or acute illness. This can worsen the symptoms and delay healing.

Sensory Impairments

Patients with sensory impairments, such as numbness or reduced sensation, should avoid moxibustion. This is because they may not be able to feel if the moxa is too hot or if the skin is becoming irritated.

Pregnancy

Moxibustion should be used with caution in pregnant women. While moxibustion can be a safe and effective treatment option for certain conditions during pregnancy, it is important to consult with a qualified practitioner and follow proper safety precautions.

Chronic Medical Conditions

Patients with chronic medical conditions, such as diabetes, heart disease, or cancer, should consult with their healthcare provider before undergoing moxibustion. This is because moxibustion may interact with certain medications or worsen symptoms.

Skin Conditions

Patients with certain skin conditions, such as eczema or psoriasis, should avoid moxibustion on the affected areas. This is because moxibustion can worsen skin irritation or trigger a flare-up.

Medical Devices

Patients with certain medical devices, such as pacemakers, should avoid moxibustion. This is because moxibustion can interfere with the function of the device and cause harm.

Allergies

Patients with allergies to mugwort or other herbs used in moxibustion should avoid this treatment. This is because it can trigger an allergic reaction, which can be severe in some cases.

It is important for patients to inform their practitioner of any health conditions, medications, or allergies they may have before undergoing moxibustion. This will help ensure that the treatment is safe and effective for them. Additionally, patients should always follow proper safety precautions, such as monitoring the temperature of the moxa and avoiding sensitive areas of the body, to minimize the risk of adverse effects.

Chapter Nine

Tips for Safe Practice

Moxibustion is a traditional Chinese medicine technique that involves the burning of dried mugwort on specific acupuncture points on the body. While moxibustion can be a safe and effective treatment option for many conditions, it is important to follow proper safety precautions to minimize the risk of adverse effects. Here are some tips for safe practice when performing moxibustion:

Use High-Quality Materials

It is important to use high-quality materials, such as dried mugwort and moxa sticks, when performing moxibustion. This will help ensure that the treatment is safe and effective.

Follow Proper Hygiene Procedures

It is important to follow proper hygiene procedures when performing moxibustion. This includes washing your hands before and after the treatment, as well as cleaning the skin and acupuncture points with alcohol before applying the moxa.

Monitor the Temperature

It is important to monitor the temperature of the moxa during the treatment. This can be done by holding the moxa close to your skin to ensure that it is not too hot. If the moxa feels too hot, you should move it away from your skin or blow on it to cool it down.

Avoid Sensitive Areas

It is important to avoid sensitive areas of the body, such as the face, genitals, and areas with thin or sensitive skin, when performing moxibustion. This will help minimize the risk of skin irritation or burns.

Use Caution with Patients with Certain Conditions

Patients with certain medical conditions, such as diabetes or heart disease, should be treated with caution when performing moxibustion. It is important to consult with a qualified practitioner and follow proper safety precautions to minimize the risk of adverse effects.

Use Caution with Pregnant Women

Moxibustion can be a safe and effective treatment option for certain conditions during pregnancy, but it is important to use caution and follow proper safety precautions. Pregnant women should consult with a qualified practitioner and avoid moxibustion on sensitive areas of the body, such as the abdomen and lower back.

Use Caution with Children and Elderly Patients

Children and elderly patients should be treated with caution when performing moxibustion. It is important to use low-temperature moxa and avoid sensitive areas of the body to minimize the risk of adverse effects.

Use Caution with Patients with Allergies

Patients with allergies to mugwort or other herbs used in moxibustion should avoid this treatment. It is important to ask patients about any allergies they may have before performing moxibustion.

Follow Proper Disposal Procedures

It is important to follow proper disposal procedures when disposing of used moxa sticks and other materials. This can help prevent fires and ensure that the environment is safe and clean.

Learning Moxibustion: Training and Certification

Moxibustion is a traditional Chinese medicine technique that involves the burning of dried mugwort on specific acupuncture points on the body. While moxibustion can be a safe and effective treatment option for many conditions, it is important for practitioners to receive proper training and certification in order to perform this technique safely and effectively.

Training in moxibustion typically involves a combination of theoretical and practical components. Theoretical components may include learning about the history and principles of moxibustion, as well as the different types of moxibustion techniques and their applications. Practical components may involve learning how to identify acupuncture points and how to perform moxibustion using different tools and materials.

There are many different organizations and institutions that offer training in moxibustion, including acupuncture schools, traditional Chinese medicine schools, and independent training centers. When choosing a training program, it is important to research the program's reputation, curriculum, and accreditation status to ensure that it meets industry standards.

In addition to formal training programs, many practitioners may also pursue certification in moxibustion through industry organizations such as the National Certification Commission for Acupuncture and Oriental Medicine (NCCAOM) in the United States. Certification typically involves passing a written exam and demonstrating proficiency in practical skills related to moxibustion.

While certification is not required in all countries, it can be a valuable credential for practitioners who wish to demonstrate their knowledge and expertise in moxibustion. It may also be required by certain regulatory bodies or insurance providers in some countries.

Practitioners should also be aware of the legal and regulatory requirements related to moxibustion in their country or region. In some countries, moxibustion may be regulated as a form of acupuncture or traditional Chinese medicine, and practitioners may be required to hold a license or certification in these fields in order to legally perform moxibustion.

In addition to formal training and certification, ongoing education and professional development can be important for practitioners who wish to continue learning and improving their skills in moxibustion. This may include attending workshops, conferences, or continuing education courses, as well as reading professional literature and keeping up with the latest research in the field.

Finding a Qualified Practitioner

Moxibustion is a traditional Chinese medicine technique that can be a safe and effective treatment option for a variety of conditions. However, it is important to find a qualified practitioner who has received proper training and certification in order to ensure that the treatment is performed safely and effectively.

One of the first steps in finding a qualified moxibustion practitioner is to research local practitioners and their credentials. This can involve checking online directories, contacting professional organizations such as the National Certification Commission for Acupuncture and Oriental Medicine (NCCAOM) or the World Federation of Acupuncture-Moxibustion Societies (WFAS), and asking for referrals from friends, family members, or healthcare providers.

Once a list of potential practitioners has been compiled, it is important to schedule a consultation or interview with each practitioner to discuss their qualifications, experience, and approach to treatment. Some key questions to ask may include:

What is your training and certification in moxibustion?

How many years of experience do you have practicing moxibustion?

What conditions do you typically treat with moxibustion?

How do you customize treatments to meet each patient's individual needs?

What are your policies on informed consent, confidentiality, and patient safety?

During the consultation or interview, it is also important to pay attention to the practitioner's communication style, demeanor, and overall professionalism. A good moxibustion practitioner should be able to establish a comfortable and trusting relationship with their patients, listen attentively to their concerns and needs, and explain the treatment process in a clear and understandable way.

In addition to finding a qualified practitioner, it is important for patients to be informed and involved in their own healthcare. This may involve doing research on the conditions being treated and the treatment options available, asking questions during consultations or appointments, and following any self-care instructions or recommendations provided by the practitioner.

Patients should also be aware of any potential risks or side effects associated with moxibustion, and should inform the practitioner of any pre-existing medical conditions, medications, or allergies before starting treatment.

Educational Programs and Requirements

Moxibustion is a traditional Chinese medicine technique that has gained popularity in recent years due to its effectiveness in treating a variety of conditions. As interest in moxibustion continues to grow, so too has the demand for educational programs and training for practitioners.

In order to become a qualified moxibustion practitioner, individuals typically need to complete a comprehensive education and training program. These programs can vary in length and scope, but generally involve coursework in traditional Chinese medicine theory, acupuncture, and moxibustion techniques and applications.

Many educational programs for moxibustion practitioners are offered by colleges and universities that specialize in traditional Chinese medicine. These programs may offer certificate, diploma, or degree options, and typically require a combination of classroom instruction, hands-on training, and clinical practice.

In addition to coursework in traditional Chinese medicine theory and moxibustion techniques, educational programs for moxibustion practitioners may also cover topics such as:

Anatomy and physiology

Acupuncture and meridian theory

Herbal medicine and nutrition

Diagnosis and treatment planning

Patient communication and ethics

Some programs may also offer specialized training in specific areas of moxibustion, such as direct or indirect techniques, or in treating specific conditions such as pain, digestive disorders, or women's health.

In addition to completing an educational program, individuals who wish to become moxibustion practitioners may also need to meet certain licensing or certification requirements. These requirements can vary depending on the state or country in which the practitioner will be practicing, and may involve passing a licensing exam or obtaining certification from a professional organization such as the NCCAOM or WFAS.

It is important for individuals who are considering a career in moxibustion to carefully research educational programs and requirements in order to ensure that they receive proper training and are able to practice safely and effectively. Some key considerations when evaluating educational programs for moxibustion practitioners may include:

1. Accreditation: Does the program have accreditation from a reputable accrediting agency, such as the Accreditation Commission for Acupuncture and Oriental Medicine (ACAOM)?

2. Curriculum: Does the program cover the necessary coursework and hands-on training required to become a competent moxibustion practitioner?

3. Faculty and resources: Does the program have experienced and knowledgeable faculty members, as well as access to the resources and facilities needed to provide quality education and training?

4. Professional development opportunities: Does the program offer opportunities for continuing education or professional development to keep up with advances in the field of moxibustion?

By carefully evaluating educational programs and requirements for moxibustion practitioners, individuals can ensure that they receive the training and credentials needed to provide safe and effective treatments to their patients.

Professional Associations and Resources

Moxibustion is an ancient traditional Chinese medicine technique that has been used for thousands of years to treat various health conditions. Moxibustion involves burning dried mugwort (Artemisia vulgaris) near specific acupoints on the body to stimulate the flow of Qi, or vital energy, in the body. As with any alternative medicine technique, it is essential to seek treatment from a qualified practitioner who has undergone extensive training and certification in the use of moxibustion.

One of the best ways to find a qualified practitioner of moxibustion is to look for professional associations and resources in your area. These organizations provide information on certified practitioners, as well as training and education programs for individuals interested in pursuing a career in moxibustion.

One such organization is the National Certification Commission for Acupuncture and Oriental Medicine (NCCAOM), which is the leading organization for certification and regulation of acupuncture and Oriental medicine in the United States. The NCCAOM offers certification for acupuncturists, herbalists, and Asian bodywork therapists, including moxibustion practitioners. To become certified by the NCCAOM, an individual must complete an accredited program of Oriental medicine, pass a comprehensive exam, and adhere to a strict code of ethics.

Another valuable resource for finding a qualified moxibustion practitioner is the American Association of Acupuncture and Oriental Medicine

(AAAOM). The AAAOM is a professional organization that promotes the integration of acupuncture and Oriental medicine into the mainstream healthcare system. The AAAOM provides a directory of certified practitioners, as well as information on educational programs and industry news.

It is also important to consider the credentials and experience of a potential moxibustion practitioner before seeking treatment. Look for practitioners who have received formal training and certification in moxibustion from accredited institutions, and who have experience treating the specific health condition you are seeking treatment for. Ask for references or testimonials from previous patients and ensure that the practitioner is licensed to practice in your state.

In addition to professional associations and resources, there are also a variety of online resources available for individuals interested in learning more about moxibustion. These resources may include educational videos, books, and articles on the history, principles, and techniques of moxibustion. It is important to note, however, that while online resources can provide valuable information, they should not be used as a substitute for professional training and certification.

Chapter Ten

Moxibustion in the Modern World

Moxibustion is an ancient healing practice that has been used in Traditional Chinese Medicine for thousands of years. However, despite its long history, moxibustion is still relevant in the modern world, and is growing in popularity as a complementary therapy alongside conventional medicine.

One reason for the continued relevance of moxibustion is its effectiveness in treating a wide range of conditions. Moxibustion is particularly effective in treating musculoskeletal conditions, such as chronic pain, arthritis, and sports injuries. It can also be used to boost the immune system, improve digestion, and regulate the menstrual cycle.

Another reason for the continued popularity of moxibustion is its safety and minimal side effects. When practiced by a qualified practitioner, moxibustion is a safe and non-invasive therapy that can be used alongside other conventional treatments.

In recent years, moxibustion has also gained recognition from the medical community as a valid complementary therapy. A growing number of hospitals and clinics now offer moxibustion alongside other conventional treatments, and more research is being conducted into its effectiveness and mechanisms of action.

As moxibustion gains wider acceptance, more people are seeking out qualified practitioners and educational programs to learn how to practice moxibustion themselves. Professional associations and resources are also becoming more available, providing a platform for practitioners to share knowledge and experiences, and to advocate for the integration of moxibustion into mainstream healthcare.

One of the challenges facing moxibustion in the modern world is the lack of regulation and standardization of training programs and practitioner qualifications. However, efforts are being made to address this issue, with organizations such as the National Certification Commission for Acupuncture and Oriental Medicine (NCCAOM) providing certification for practitioners of moxibustion and other Traditional Chinese Medicine therapies.

Another challenge is the need for more research into the effectiveness of moxibustion and its mechanisms of action. While there is a growing body of research into moxibustion, more studies are needed to fully understand its effects and to determine the best conditions for its use.

Despite these challenges, moxibustion continues to be a valuable and effective healing practice in the modern world. As more people discover the benefits of moxibustion and seek out qualified practitioners, the integration of moxibustion into mainstream healthcare is likely to continue. With ongoing research and efforts to standardize training and qualifications, moxibustion has the potential to become an even more widely accepted and utilized therapy in the years to come.

Current Research and Developments

Moxibustion is a traditional Chinese medicine technique that has been used for thousands of years to treat a variety of health conditions. It involves burning dried mugwort (Artemisia vulgaris) on or near the skin at specific acupoints on the body. Moxibustion is believed to work by stimulating the flow of Qi, or vital energy, throughout the body, which can help to restore balance and promote healing.

In recent years, there has been a growing interest in the use of moxibustion in the Western world, and a number of studies have been conducted to investigate its effectiveness and safety. Here, we will explore some of the current research and developments in the field of moxibustion.

One area of interest for researchers has been the use of moxibustion for pain management. A study published in the Journal of Acupuncture and Meridian Studies found that moxibustion was effective in reducing pain and inflammation in patients with knee osteoarthritis. Another study published in the Journal of Alternative and Complementary Medicine found that moxibustion was effective in reducing pain and improving function in patients with chronic low back pain.

Other studies have explored the use of moxibustion for digestive disorders. A study published in the World Journal of Gastroenterology found that moxibustion was effective in reducing symptoms of irritable bowel syndrome. Another study published in the Journal of Traditional Chinese Medicine found that moxibustion was effective in treating gastroesophageal reflux disease.

There has also been interest in the use of moxibustion for women's health issues, such as menstrual pain and infertility. A study published in the Journal of Acupuncture and Meridian Studies found that moxibustion was effective in reducing menstrual pain. Another study published in the Journal of Traditional Chinese Medicine found that moxibustion was effective in improving pregnancy rates in women undergoing in vitro fertilization.

In addition to its use in specific health conditions, researchers have also explored the broader applications of moxibustion for promoting overall wellness. A study published in the Journal of Traditional Chinese Medicine found that moxibustion was effective in reducing stress and improving immune function in healthy individuals.

While there is promising research on the effectiveness of moxibustion, there are also ongoing efforts to further understand its mechanisms of action and improve its delivery. One area of development has been the use of moxibustion in conjunction with modern medical technologies, such as magnetic resonance imaging (MRI). A study published in the Journal of Magnetic Resonance Imaging found that moxibustion produced distinct neural activity in the brain that could be observed on MRI scans.

Another area of development has been the refinement of moxibustion techniques and materials. For example, a study published in the Journal of Acupuncture and Meridian Studies found that a new type of smokeless moxa stick was effective in delivering heat to acupoints without producing smoke or odor.

Integrating Moxibustion into Western Medicine

Integrating Moxibustion into Western Medicine

Moxibustion, a traditional Chinese medicine therapy that uses burning of moxa (dried mugwort herb) to stimulate acupoints on the body, has been practiced for thousands of years in China and other Asian countries. In recent years, there has been a growing interest in integrating moxibustion into Western medicine as a complementary therapy for various conditions. Below we will discuss the benefits and challenges of integrating moxibustion into Western medicine and the current research and developments in this field.

Benefits of Integrating Moxibustion into Western Medicine:

Moxibustion has been found to be effective in treating a wide range of conditions, including pain, digestive disorders, respiratory issues, women's health, and many others. It has also been found to be safe and well-tolerated when performed by a qualified practitioner. Integrating moxibustion into Western medicine has several benefits, including:

1. Complementary Therapy: Moxibustion can be used as a complementary therapy to Western medicine, which can enhance the effectiveness of treatment and improve patient outcomes. For example, moxibustion can be used to manage pain and reduce the need for pain medications.

2. Cost-effective: Moxibustion is a cost-effective therapy that can reduce healthcare costs. In some cases, moxibustion can be used as an alternative to more expensive Western medical treatments.

3. Patient-centered Care: Integrating moxibustion into Western medicine can provide a more patient-centered approach to care. Patients can have a choice of treatments that are safe, effective, and aligned with their beliefs and preferences.

Challenges of Integrating Moxibustion into Western Medicine:

Despite the potential benefits of integrating moxibustion into Western medicine, there are several challenges that need to be addressed:

4. Lack of Standardization: Moxibustion is a complex therapy that requires extensive training and experience. There is a lack of standardization in the practice of moxibustion, which makes it difficult to ensure quality and safety.

5. Limited Research: There is limited research on the effectiveness of moxibustion, which makes it difficult to determine its benefits and risks. More high-quality research is needed to establish the efficacy of moxibustion for various conditions.

6. Integration with Western Medical Practice: Integrating moxibustion into Western medicine requires collaboration between practitioners of traditional Chinese medicine and Western medicine. This can be challenging due to differences in philosophy, training, and practice.

Current Research and Developments:

Despite the challenges, there is a growing interest in integrating moxibustion into Western medicine, and several studies have been conducted to investigate its effectiveness. For example, a systematic review and meta-analysis published in the Journal of Pain in 2017 found that moxibustion was effective in reducing chronic low back pain. Another study published in the Journal of Alternative and Complementary Medicine in 2019 found that moxibustion combined with acupuncture was effective in treating post-stroke depression.

There are also ongoing efforts to standardize the practice of moxibustion and to integrate it into Western medical practice. The World Health Organization (WHO) has recognized moxibustion as a complementary therapy and has published guidelines for its safe and effective use. In addition, several professional associations, such as the American Society of Acupuncturists and the National Certification Commission for Acupuncture and Oriental Medicine, have established standards for the practice of moxibustion.

The Future of Moxibustion

Moxibustion has a rich history that dates back over 2,500 years in Traditional Chinese Medicine. Over the years, it has become more popular in Western countries, with practitioners and patients alike finding it to be a valuable complementary therapy. As research on the benefits of moxibustion continues to grow, the future of this practice looks promising.

One area that could see growth in the future is the integration of moxibustion into mainstream Western medicine. While acupuncture has become more accepted in Western medicine, moxibustion is still considered an alternative therapy. However, as more studies show the efficacy of moxibustion, it is possible that it could become a more commonly recommended treatment for certain conditions.

Another area of potential growth is the development of new techniques and technologies for moxibustion. While the basic principles and tools of moxibustion have remained the same for centuries, there is always room for innovation and improvement. For example, some practitioners are exploring the use of moxibustion in conjunction with other therapies, such as massage and cupping, to enhance the overall effects.

In addition, there is ongoing research into the mechanisms of moxibustion and how it affects the body. This could lead to a better understanding of how moxibustion works and how it can be optimized for specific conditions. For example, some studies have looked at the effects of moxibustion on the immune system, and there may be potential for using moxibustion to support the body's natural defenses against illness.

The future of moxibustion may also include further development of educational programs and resources for practitioners. As moxibustion becomes more popular, there may be a need for more standardized training and certification programs to ensure that practitioners are properly trained and qualified to provide safe and effective treatments.

Chapter Eleven

Moxibustion for Emotional Well-being

Moxibustion is a traditional Chinese medicine therapy that uses heat to stimulate acupoints on the body. This therapy has been used for thousands of years to treat a variety of physical ailments and conditions, but it is also gaining recognition as a way to improve emotional well-being.

Emotional well-being is an important aspect of overall health, and it can be affected by a variety of factors, including stress, anxiety, depression, and other mental health conditions. Moxibustion has been found to be effective in helping to alleviate some of these emotional issues.

One of the ways that moxibustion can help improve emotional well-being is by reducing stress. When a person is under stress, their body produces cortisol, a hormone that can cause inflammation and other negative effects. Moxibustion has been found to lower cortisol levels, which can help reduce stress and its negative effects on the body.

Moxibustion has also been found to be effective in treating anxiety and depression. One study found that patients with anxiety who received moxibustion therapy experienced a significant reduction in their symptoms compared to those who did not receive the therapy. Another study found that moxibustion was effective in treating depression and was able to increase the levels of serotonin and dopamine in the body, which are chemicals that help regulate mood.

In addition to reducing stress, anxiety, and depression, moxibustion can also help improve sleep quality. Poor sleep is often associated with emotional issues, and moxibustion has been found to improve sleep quality by promoting relaxation and reducing stress levels.

Moxibustion can also help improve digestion, which can have a positive effect on emotional well-being. The gut-brain axis is a complex system that connects the digestive system and the brain, and research has found that changes in the gut microbiome can affect mood and behavior. Moxibustion has been found to improve digestion and balance the gut microbiome, which can have a positive effect on emotional health.

There are several acupoints that are commonly used in moxibustion therapy to improve emotional well-being. The Shenmen point, located on the wrist, is commonly used to reduce anxiety and promote relaxation. The Neiguan point, located on the inside of the wrist, is used to reduce stress and improve digestion. The Zusanli point, located on the lower leg, is used to promote relaxation and reduce stress.

It is important to note that moxibustion should not be used as a sole treatment for emotional issues. It is important to seek the guidance of a trained practitioner who can recommend the best course of treatment based on individual needs and circumstances.

Balancing Emotions

Moxibustion is a traditional Chinese medicine practice that uses burning mugwort (Artemisia vulgaris) on or near specific acupuncture points to stimulate healing in the body. It has been used for thousands of years to treat a variety of physical and mental health conditions. One of the benefits of moxibustion is that it can be used to balance emotions and improve overall emotional well-being.

According to traditional Chinese medicine, emotions are closely tied to the body's internal organs and their corresponding meridians. When there is an imbalance or blockage in the flow of energy (Qi) through these meridians, emotions can become imbalanced as well. Moxibustion can help to restore the flow of Qi and balance emotions.

There are several acupuncture points that are commonly used in moxibustion for emotional well-being. These include the Conception Vessel 17 (CV17) point, also known as the "Sea of Tranquility," which is located in the center of the chest and is believed to calm the mind and regulate emotions. The Pericardium 6 (PC6) point, located on the inside of the wrist, is another commonly used point for emotional balance and can help to alleviate anxiety and stress. The Kidney 3 (KI3) point, located on the inner ankle, is also believed to help balance emotions and promote calmness.

In addition to these specific acupuncture points, moxibustion can be used to balance emotions by addressing imbalances in the body as a whole. For example, if someone is experiencing feelings of anger or frustration, moxibustion may be applied to the Liver meridian to help clear any blockages and restore balance to the body.

Moxibustion can also be used in combination with other therapies to enhance emotional well-being. For example, it can be used in conjunction with acupuncture, massage therapy, or counseling to provide a comprehensive approach to emotional healing. Moxibustion can also be used in combination with herbal remedies to support overall emotional balance.

Research has shown that moxibustion can be effective in improving emotional well-being. A study published in the Journal of Alternative and Complementary Medicine found that moxibustion was effective in reducing symptoms of depression and anxiety in patients with chronic obstructive pulmonary disease (COPD). Another study published in the Journal of Traditional Chinese Medicine found that moxibustion was effective in improving emotional well-being and overall quality of life in patients with Parkinson's disease.

It is important to note that while moxibustion can be a helpful tool in promoting emotional balance, it is not a substitute for professional mental health treatment. Anyone experiencing severe or persistent emotional symptoms should seek the guidance of a licensed mental health professional.

Moxibustion for Stress and Anxiety

Moxibustion, an ancient Chinese therapy, has been used for centuries to promote healing and improve overall health. It involves the burning of dried mugwort, also known as moxa, at specific acupuncture points to stimulate the flow of energy, or qi, in the body. Moxibustion is believed to have a number of health benefits, including reducing stress and anxiety. Below we will explore how moxibustion can be used as a therapy for stress and anxiety, and the research that supports its effectiveness.

Stress and anxiety are common problems in modern society, affecting millions of people worldwide. These conditions can cause a range of physical and mental symptoms, including muscle tension, headaches, fatigue, irritability, and difficulty concentrating. Chronic stress and anxiety can have long-term effects on both physical and mental health, increasing the risk of heart disease, stroke, depression, and other conditions.

Moxibustion is believed to be an effective therapy for stress and anxiety, as it helps to calm the mind and promote relaxation. The therapy works by activating specific acupuncture points, which in turn stimulate the release of endorphins, the body's natural painkillers. Endorphins also have a calming effect on the mind, reducing feelings of stress and anxiety.

In addition, moxibustion has been shown to regulate the autonomic nervous system, which plays a key role in stress responses. The therapy is believed to help balance the sympathetic and parasympathetic nervous systems, which control the "fight or flight" response and the "rest and digest" response, respectively. By balancing these systems, moxibustion can help reduce the physical symptoms of stress and anxiety, such as rapid heartbeat and shallow breathing.

Research has shown that moxibustion can be an effective therapy for stress and anxiety. In a study published in the Journal of Acupuncture and Meridian Studies, researchers found that moxibustion significantly reduced symptoms of anxiety in participants with chronic obstructive pulmonary disease (COPD). The therapy was also found to improve quality of life and reduce the need for medication in these patients.

Another study, published in the Journal of Alternative and Complementary Medicine, found that moxibustion significantly reduced symptoms of anxiety and depression in participants with irritable bowel syndrome (IBS). The therapy was also found to improve overall quality of life and reduce the severity of IBS symptoms.

Moxibustion can be used alone or in combination with other therapies, such as acupuncture, massage, and herbal medicine, to treat stress and anxiety. The therapy can be performed by a qualified practitioner, who will carefully select acupuncture points based on the individual's specific needs and symptoms. Moxibustion can also be performed at home using moxa sticks, which are readily available at health food stores and online.

It is important to note that moxibustion should not be used as a substitute for conventional medical care for stress and anxiety. It is always recommended to consult with a healthcare professional before starting any new therapy, especially if you have a medical condition or are taking medication.

In addition, moxibustion is generally considered safe when performed by a qualified practitioner. However, there are some precautions that should be taken to ensure the safety of the therapy. For example, moxibustion should not be performed on areas of the skin that are inflamed, infected, or have open wounds. It should also be avoided in individuals with certain medical conditions, such as pregnancy, epilepsy, and certain types of cancer.

Moxibustion for Depression

Moxibustion is an alternative therapy that has been used for centuries in traditional Chinese medicine. It involves the burning of mugwort, a type of herb, to stimulate acupoints on the body. While often used for physical conditions, moxibustion can also be used to treat emotional disorders, such as depression. Below we will explore the use of moxibustion for depression and how it may benefit individuals struggling with this mental health condition.

Depression is a common mental health condition that affects millions of people worldwide. Symptoms can include persistent sadness, lack of energy, difficulty concentrating, and feelings of worthlessness. Traditional treatments for depression often include medication, talk therapy, or a combination of both. However, some individuals may be hesitant to try traditional methods or may not find them effective. This is where alternative therapies, such as moxibustion, can come into play.

Moxibustion for depression involves the stimulation of acupoints on the body with the burning of mugwort. Mugwort is thought to have a warming effect on the body, which can help to improve circulation and promote relaxation. Acupoints that are targeted for depression include those that are associated with the liver, spleen, and kidney. These organs are believed to play a role in regulating mood and emotions.

Studies have shown that moxibustion can be effective in reducing symptoms of depression. One study conducted in China found that individuals who received moxibustion in addition to their traditional treatment had significantly lower depression scores compared to those who only received traditional treatment. Another study found that moxibustion was effective in improving both physical and mental symptoms of depression.

While the exact mechanism of how moxibustion works for depression is not fully understood, it is thought to involve the release of endorphins, which are natural painkillers produced by the body. Endorphins can help to reduce feelings of pain and increase feelings of pleasure and happiness. Additionally, moxibustion may also help to regulate levels of neurotransmitters, such as serotonin and dopamine, which are known to play a role in mood and emotions.

It is important to note that moxibustion should not be used as a replacement for traditional treatments for depression. It is best used as a complementary therapy, in addition to other treatments prescribed by a healthcare professional. Moxibustion should also be performed by a trained practitioner to ensure safety and effectiveness.

In addition to moxibustion, there are other alternative therapies that can be used to help with depression. Acupuncture, for example, involves the insertion of thin needles into specific acupoints on the body to stimulate the flow of energy. Like moxibustion, acupuncture has been found to be effective in reducing symptoms of depression.

Other alternative therapies that may be beneficial for depression include massage therapy, aromatherapy, and meditation. Massage therapy involves the manipulation of soft tissues in the body to promote relaxation and reduce stress. Aromatherapy involves the use of essential oils, which are thought to have therapeutic properties that can help to improve mood and reduce stress. Meditation involves the practice of mindfulness and can help to reduce feelings of anxiety and depression.

Chapter Twelve

Moxibustion for Sleep

Moxibustion is a traditional Chinese medicine therapy that involves the burning of mugwort herb, also known as moxa, to stimulate specific acupuncture points on the body. This therapy has been used for centuries to treat a variety of health conditions and is believed to help balance the body's energy, or qi, and promote healing.

One of the health conditions that can be treated with moxibustion is sleep disorders. Insomnia is a common problem that affects many people and can lead to a variety of health issues, including fatigue, irritability, and decreased cognitive function. Moxibustion can help to promote relaxation and reduce stress, which can lead to improved sleep.

Moxibustion works by stimulating the acupuncture points that are associated with sleep. One of these points is called the Shenmen point, which is located on the wrist. This point is associated with the heart and can help to calm the mind and promote relaxation. By stimulating this point with moxibustion, it is possible to promote relaxation and reduce stress, which can lead to improved sleep.

Another point that can be stimulated with moxibustion to improve sleep is the Anmian point, which is located behind the ear. This point is associated with the nervous system and can help to promote relaxation and reduce tension. By stimulating this point with moxibustion, it is possible to promote relaxation and reduce stress, which can lead to improved sleep.

Moxibustion can also be used to treat other sleep disorders, such as sleep apnea. This condition is characterized by pauses in breathing during sleep, which can lead to snoring and daytime fatigue. Moxibustion can help to improve respiratory function and promote relaxation, which can reduce the symptoms of sleep apnea.

In addition to promoting relaxation and reducing stress, moxibustion can also help to regulate the body's circadian rhythms, which can improve sleep quality. Circadian rhythms are the body's natural cycles that regulate sleep, wakefulness, and other physiological processes. By promoting the balance of these rhythms, moxibustion can help to improve sleep quality and promote overall health.

It is important to note that moxibustion should be performed by a qualified practitioner to ensure safety and effectiveness. The practitioner will determine the appropriate acupuncture points to stimulate based on the individual's specific needs and health conditions.

In addition to moxibustion, other natural remedies can also be used to promote sleep, including aromatherapy and herbal medicine. Lavender essential oil, for example, is known for its calming properties and can be used to promote relaxation and reduce anxiety. Chamomile tea is also a natural remedy that can be used to promote relaxation and improve sleep quality.

Insomnia and Sleep Disorders

Insomnia is a sleep disorder that is characterized by difficulty falling asleep, staying asleep, or both. It is a common condition affecting millions of people worldwide, and if left untreated, it can lead to serious health problems. Moxibustion, a traditional Chinese medicine practice, has been used for centuries to treat insomnia and other sleep disorders. Below we will explore the use of moxibustion in treating insomnia and sleep disorders, how it works, and its benefits.

Moxibustion is a type of therapy that involves burning dried mugwort (also known as moxa) to stimulate acupoints on the body. This therapy is believed to help regulate the flow of energy (known as qi) in the body, thereby restoring balance and promoting healing. The use of moxibustion for insomnia and sleep disorders is based on the principles of traditional Chinese medicine, which views sleep as an essential component of good health and well-being.

According to traditional Chinese medicine, insomnia and sleep disorders are caused by imbalances in the body's energy, particularly the liver and heart meridians. The liver meridian is responsible for regulating emotions and stress, while the heart meridian governs sleep and consciousness. When there is an imbalance in these meridians, it can lead to insomnia, anxiety, and other sleep disorders.

Moxibustion is believed to work by restoring balance to these meridians and promoting relaxation. The heat generated by burning the moxa is said to penetrate deep into the body, stimulating the acupoints and increasing blood flow. This, in turn, is thought to promote the release of natural painkillers and other chemicals that help the body to relax and unwind.

Studies have shown that moxibustion can be an effective treatment for insomnia and other sleep disorders. One study published in the Journal of Traditional Chinese Medicine found that moxibustion combined with acupuncture was effective in treating insomnia in elderly patients. Another study published in the Journal of Sleep Research found that moxibustion was effective in improving sleep quality in patients with chronic obstructive pulmonary disease (COPD).

Moxibustion is also believed to have other benefits for sleep, including reducing anxiety and promoting relaxation. According to a review of studies published in the Journal of Acupuncture and Meridian Studies, moxibustion was effective in reducing anxiety in patients with anxiety disorders. The review also found that moxibustion had a calming effect on the nervous system, which may help to promote relaxation and improve sleep quality.

Moxibustion is a safe and non-invasive therapy that can be used alone or in combination with other treatments for insomnia and sleep disorders. It is generally well-tolerated, although some people may experience mild discomfort or skin irritation at the site of the moxibustion. It is important to seek treatment from a qualified practitioner who can ensure that the therapy is administered safely and effectively.

In addition to moxibustion, there are other natural remedies and lifestyle changes that can help to improve sleep quality and reduce the symptoms of insomnia and sleep disorders. These include:

1. Establishing a regular sleep routine: Going to bed and waking up at the same time every day can help to regulate the body's natural sleep-wake cycle and promote better sleep.

2. Creating a comfortable sleep environment: Make sure your bedroom is cool, quiet, and dark, and invest in a comfortable mattress and pillows.

3. Avoiding caffeine and alcohol: These substances can interfere with sleep quality and make it harder to fall asleep.

4. Practicing relaxation techniques: Deep breathing, meditation, and yoga can help to reduce stress and promote relaxation.

5. Getting regular exercise: Exercise can help to promote better sleep, but it is important to avoid exercising too

Establishing Healthy Sleep Patterns

Establishing Healthy Sleep Patterns

Sleep is an essential component of human life, and it is important to establish healthy sleep patterns to ensure that our bodies and minds can function optimally. Unfortunately, many people struggle with sleep-related issues, such as insomnia, sleep apnea, and restless leg syndrome. These conditions can significantly affect one's quality of life, making it difficult to focus during the day and leading to feelings of exhaustion and irritability. While there are many treatments available for sleep disorders, some people turn to alternative therapies such as moxibustion to help establish healthy sleep patterns.

Moxibustion is an ancient Chinese therapy that involves the burning of dried mugwort (Artemisia vulgaris) on specific acupuncture points on the body. It is believed to help promote the flow of Qi (pronounced "chee"), or life force, throughout the body, which can help to restore balance and promote healing. Moxibustion has been used for thousands of years to treat a wide range of health issues, including sleep disorders.

There are several acupuncture points on the body that are thought to be particularly effective for promoting healthy sleep patterns. One of the most commonly used points is known as Shenmen, which translates to "spirit gate" in Chinese. This point is located on the inside of the wrist, and it is believed to help calm the mind and reduce feelings of anxiety and stress, which can be major contributors to insomnia.

Another commonly used point for sleep disorders is known as Yin Tang, which is located between the eyebrows. This point is believed to help regulate the body's natural sleep-wake cycle and promote relaxation, making it easier to fall asleep and stay asleep throughout the night.

1. Moxibustion is typically administered in one of two ways: direct or indirect. Direct moxibustion involves placing a small amount of dried mugwort directly on the skin and lighting it, allowing it to burn down until it is extinguished. Indirect moxibustion involves burning the mugwort on a piece of ginger, garlic, or other substances that are placed on the skin. The heat from the burning mugwort penetrates the skin and stimulates the acupuncture point, helping to promote healing and restore balance to the body.

In addition to moxibustion, there are several other things that people can do to establish healthy sleep patterns. One of the most important is to establish a regular sleep routine, which involves going to bed and waking up at the same time each day. This can help to regulate the body's natural sleep-wake cycle and make it easier to fall asleep and stay asleep throughout the night.

It is also important to create a sleep-conducive environment, which includes keeping the bedroom dark, cool, and quiet. Avoiding electronics such as smartphones, tablets, and televisions before bedtime can also be helpful, as the blue light emitted by these devices can interfere with the body's natural sleep-wake cycle.

Exercise and diet can also play a role in promoting healthy sleep patterns. Regular exercise has been shown to improve the quality of sleep, while a diet rich in fruits, vegetables, and whole grains can help to regulate the body's natural sleep-wake cycle.

Moxibustion for Restorative Sleep

Moxibustion is an ancient Chinese therapy that involves the burning of the mugwort herb to stimulate acupuncture points on the body. It is often used as a complementary therapy to acupuncture, but can also be used on its own. One of the potential benefits of moxibustion is its ability to promote restorative sleep.

Restorative sleep is important for overall health and well-being. It is during this stage of sleep that the body repairs and regenerates tissues, strengthens the immune system, and consolidates memories. Without restorative sleep, individuals may experience fatigue, cognitive impairment, and a weakened immune system.

Moxibustion can be used to promote restorative sleep by stimulating specific acupuncture points on the body that are associated with sleep and relaxation. One such point is the Shenmen, also known as the "Spirit Gate," which is located on the wrist. Stimulating this point with moxibustion can help to calm the mind and promote relaxation.

Another point that is commonly used for sleep issues is the Anmian, which is located behind the ear. Stimulating this point with moxibustion has been shown to improve sleep quality and duration.

Moxibustion can also be used to promote restorative sleep by addressing underlying health issues that may be contributing to sleep disturbances. For example, moxibustion can be used to stimulate points associated with digestion and the liver, which can help to alleviate insomnia related to digestive issues or stress.

Moxibustion can also be used to address imbalances in the body's energy, or qi, that may be contributing to sleep disturbances. For example, if an individual has a deficiency of qi, they may experience fatigue and difficulty falling asleep. Moxibustion can be used to stimulate specific points to improve the flow of qi and restore balance to the body.

In addition to moxibustion, other lifestyle changes can also be helpful in promoting restorative sleep. This may include practicing good sleep hygiene, such as establishing a consistent sleep schedule and avoiding caffeine and alcohol before bedtime. Exercise and relaxation techniques, such as yoga or meditation, may also be beneficial.

It is important to note that moxibustion should be used as part of a comprehensive treatment plan for sleep issues, and should always be performed by a qualified practitioner. Additionally, moxibustion should not be used as a substitute for medical treatment for underlying health conditions that may be contributing to sleep disturbances.

Chapter Thirteen

Moxibustion for Skin Health

Moxibustion is an ancient healing technique in traditional Chinese medicine that involves burning dried mugwort on specific points of the body. While moxibustion is commonly known for its effectiveness in treating pain and other physical ailments, it can also be used to improve skin health.

The principles of moxibustion are based on the concept of qi, the vital energy that flows through the body, and the balance of yin and yang, the opposing forces that govern the body's functions. When qi is blocked or out of balance, it can manifest as physical or emotional symptoms, including skin conditions.

Moxibustion is believed to help balance the body's energy by warming the meridians, or energy channels, and stimulating the flow of qi. This can have a positive impact on the health of the skin, which is connected to the lung and large intestine meridians.

Moxibustion can be used to treat a variety of skin conditions, including acne, eczema, psoriasis, and rosacea. It is often used in conjunction with acupuncture, herbs, and other therapies to address underlying imbalances in the body that may be contributing to skin issues.

For example, moxibustion can be used to treat acne by stimulating blood flow and reducing inflammation in the affected areas. It can also help to balance hormones and reduce stress, which can contribute to the development of acne.

Moxibustion can also be used to treat eczema, a chronic skin condition characterized by red, itchy, and inflamed patches of skin. By stimulating the flow of qi and addressing underlying imbalances, moxibustion can help to reduce inflammation and itching, as well as improve overall skin health.

In addition to treating specific skin conditions, moxibustion can also be used as a preventive measure to maintain healthy skin. Regular moxibustion treatments can help to improve circulation, boost the immune system, and promote overall health and wellness, all of which can contribute to healthy, radiant skin.

When using moxibustion for skin health, it is important to work with a qualified practitioner who can assess your individual needs and create a treatment plan tailored to your specific condition. Moxibustion should also be used in conjunction with other healthy habits, such as eating a balanced diet, staying hydrated, getting adequate sleep, and avoiding smoking and excessive alcohol consumption.

Acne and Eczema

Moxibustion is a traditional Chinese medicine therapy that involves burning dried mugwort on or near specific acupoints on the body to stimulate healing and promote balance. While many people are familiar with acupuncture, which also involves the use of acupoints, moxibustion is another effective therapy that can be used to treat a variety of conditions, including skin health issues like acne and eczema.

Acne is a common skin condition that affects millions of people worldwide. It is caused by the overproduction of sebum, an oily substance that is produced by the sebaceous glands in the skin. When the pores become clogged with sebum, dead skin cells, and bacteria, it can lead to the formation of pimples, blackheads, and whiteheads. While there are many treatments available for acne, including topical medications, oral medications, and skincare products, moxibustion is a natural and effective alternative therapy that can help to reduce inflammation, balance hormones, and improve overall skin health.

Moxibustion can be used to treat acne by targeting specific acupoints on the body that are related to skin health. For example, the acupoint known as LI4, located on the hand between the thumb and index finger, is believed to stimulate the immune system and reduce inflammation. Another acupoint, located on the face near the nose and called ST4, is believed to improve overall skin health and reduce the appearance of acne.

In addition to treating acne, moxibustion can also be used to treat eczema, a skin condition characterized by dry, itchy, and inflamed skin. Eczema can be caused by a variety of factors, including allergies, stress, and hormonal imbalances. Moxibustion can help to address these underlying causes by stimulating the body's natural healing processes and promoting balance throughout the body.

One study published in the Journal of Traditional Chinese Medicine found that moxibustion was effective in treating eczema in 76% of cases. The study involved 50 patients with chronic eczema who received moxibustion treatment twice a week for 12 weeks. The results showed significant improvements in skin condition, with a reduction in itching, redness, and inflammation.

Moxibustion works by stimulating the flow of Qi, or life force energy, throughout the body. When Qi is blocked or stagnant, it can lead to a variety of health issues, including skin problems like acne and eczema.

By targeting specific acupoints on the body with the heat and energy of burning mugwort, moxibustion can help to clear blockages and restore balance to the body.

Moxibustion is a safe and effective therapy that can be used in combination with other natural remedies and conventional treatments for skin health issues like acne and eczema. It is important to seek out a qualified and experienced practitioner who can provide guidance and support in using moxibustion as part of a comprehensive treatment plan.

In addition to moxibustion, there are other natural remedies that can be used to support healthy skin, including a balanced diet, regular exercise, stress management, and proper skincare. By taking a holistic approach to skin health, it is possible to achieve clear, healthy, and radiant skin that supports overall health and wellbeing.

Psoriasis and Skin Rashes

Psoriasis and skin rashes are common skin conditions that affect many people worldwide. While there are various treatments available, some people may turn to traditional Chinese medicine (TCM) and moxibustion as a natural and effective alternative.

Psoriasis is a chronic autoimmune condition that causes the skin cells to grow too quickly, resulting in thick, scaly patches on the skin's surface. It can affect any part of the body, including the scalp, elbows, knees, and lower back. It is a chronic condition, and while there is no cure, treatment can help manage symptoms.

Skin rashes, on the other hand, can be caused by a wide range of factors, including allergies, infections, and autoimmune diseases. They can manifest as red, itchy, and inflamed patches on the skin, and can cause discomfort and embarrassment.

Moxibustion, a traditional Chinese medicine technique, involves burning dried mugwort on or near the skin's surface to stimulate acupuncture points. This technique has been used for centuries in TCM to treat various health conditions, including skin disorders.

Moxibustion for Psoriasis

Moxibustion is believed to work for psoriasis by stimulating the immune system and reducing inflammation. It is thought to improve blood circulation, which can promote healing and reduce skin irritation.

One study published in the Journal of Traditional Chinese Medicine found that moxibustion combined with acupuncture can effectively reduce psoriasis symptoms. The study involved 50 psoriasis patients who received either acupuncture and moxibustion or traditional medication. The group that received acupuncture and moxibustion had a higher rate of improvement in symptoms, including a reduction in scaling, itching, and redness.

Another study published in the Journal of Acupuncture and Meridian Studies found that moxibustion combined with herbal medicine can improve psoriasis symptoms by regulating the immune system and reducing inflammation.

Moxibustion for Skin Rashes

Moxibustion can also be effective in treating skin rashes by improving blood circulation and reducing inflammation. It is believed to stimulate the immune system and promote the body's natural healing process.

A study published in the Journal of Traditional Chinese Medicine found that moxibustion can effectively treat eczema by reducing inflammation and itching. The study involved 70 eczema patients who received either moxibustion or traditional medication. The group that received moxibustion had a higher rate of improvement in symptoms, including a reduction in itching, redness, and inflammation.

Another study published in the Journal of Acupuncture and Meridian Studies found that moxibustion can effectively treat pruritus, a common symptom of skin rashes. The study involved 30 pruritus patients who received either moxibustion or traditional medication. The group that received moxibustion had a higher rate of improvement in symptoms, including a reduction in itching and skin irritation.

Safety Considerations

Moxibustion is generally safe when performed by a qualified practitioner. However, there are some safety considerations to keep in mind. Moxibustion should not be used on open wounds or broken skin, as it may increase the risk of infection. It should also be avoided in pregnant women and people with certain medical conditions, such as cancer or diabetes.

It is important to choose a qualified practitioner who has received proper training and certification in moxibustion. The practitioner should also follow strict hygiene practices and use sterile equipment to minimize the risk of infection.

Scar Tissue and Wound Healing

Moxibustion, a traditional Chinese medicine technique, has been used for centuries to promote wound healing and to treat scar tissue. Moxibustion uses the heat generated by burning mugwort (Artemisia vulgaris) to stimulate specific acupuncture points on the body, creating a therapeutic effect. This technique can be used on its own or in conjunction with acupuncture, massage, or other forms of therapy.

Scar tissue can form due to a variety of reasons, including injury, surgery, or inflammation. While scar tissue is an essential part of the healing process, it can sometimes be unsightly or cause discomfort. Moxibustion has been shown to be effective in reducing scar tissue and improving the appearance of scars. The heat generated by the burning mugwort helps to increase circulation to the affected area, which can promote the healing process and reduce inflammation. The increased circulation can also help to break up scar tissue and soften the skin.

Moxibustion has also been used to help promote wound healing. When applied to the skin, mugwort has been shown to have antibacterial and anti-inflammatory properties that can help prevent infection and reduce swelling. By increasing blood flow to the affected area, moxibustion can also help to speed up the healing process.

One study published in the Journal of Alternative and Complementary Medicine found that moxibustion was effective in improving wound healing in rats. The researchers found that moxibustion helped to increase blood flow to the affected area and reduce the size of the wound. Another study published in the same journal found that moxibustion was effective in reducing the size of scars in rats.

Moxibustion can be used to treat a variety of different types of scars, including keloid scars, hypertrophic scars, and atrophic scars. Keloid scars are raised, thickened scars that can be difficult to treat. Moxibustion can be used to soften the skin and reduce the size of the scar. Hypertrophic scars are similar to keloid scars but do not extend beyond the boundaries of the original wound. Moxibustion can be used to reduce the size of hypertrophic scars and improve their appearance. Atrophic scars are depressed scars that can result from acne or injury. Moxibustion can be used to increase blood flow to the affected area, which can help to improve the appearance of atrophic scars.

In addition to promoting wound healing and reducing scar tissue, moxibustion can also be used to treat a variety of skin conditions. Acne is a common skin condition that can be treated with moxibustion. The heat generated by the burning mugwort can help to reduce inflammation and kill bacteria, which can help to prevent acne breakouts. Eczema is another skin condition that can be treated with moxibustion. The heat generated by the burning mugwort can help to reduce inflammation and soothe itching.

Psoriasis is a chronic autoimmune disorder that affects the skin. While there is no cure for psoriasis, moxibustion can help to reduce the symptoms of the condition. Moxibustion can help to reduce inflammation and promote skin health, which can help to improve the appearance of psoriasis lesions. Skin rashes can also be treated with moxibustion. The heat generated by the burning mugwort can help to reduce inflammation and soothe itching.

Moxibustion is a safe and effective therapy that can be used to treat a variety of skin conditions and promote wound healing. However, there are some precautions that should be taken when using moxibustion. It is important to make sure that the practitioner is licensed and experienced in the use of moxibustion. The skin should also be protected during

Chapter Fourteen

Moxibustion for Musculoskeletal Issues

Moxibustion is an ancient form of Chinese medicine that involves the use of heat and herbs to stimulate specific acupoints on the body. This therapy has been used for thousands of years to treat a variety of conditions, including musculoskeletal issues. Below we will explore how moxibustion can be used to relieve pain, reduce inflammation, and promote healing in the muscles and joints.

Musculoskeletal issues are a common problem that can affect people of all ages. This type of issue can arise from overuse, injury, or aging. Some common musculoskeletal conditions include arthritis, back pain, neck pain, and tendonitis. While Western medicine typically treats these conditions with medication, physical therapy, and surgery, moxibustion offers an alternative treatment option that can be used alone or in conjunction with other therapies.

Moxibustion works by stimulating acupoints along the body's meridians. The heat and herbs used in this therapy help to increase blood flow to the affected area, which can promote healing and reduce pain. The use of moxibustion can also help to reduce inflammation in the muscles and joints, which can further reduce pain and improve mobility.

One of the most common uses of moxibustion for musculoskeletal issues is in the treatment of arthritis. Arthritis is a condition that causes inflammation in the joints, leading to pain, stiffness, and reduced mobility. Moxibustion can be used to reduce inflammation in the affected joints, which can help to relieve pain and improve range of motion. Additionally, the heat and herbs used in moxibustion can help to promote the production of synovial fluid, which helps to lubricate the joints and reduce friction.

Another common use of moxibustion for musculoskeletal issues is in the treatment of back pain. Back pain can be caused by a variety of factors, including muscle strain, herniated discs, and spinal stenosis. Moxibustion can be used to relax the muscles in the back, which can help to relieve pain and improve mobility. Additionally, the heat and herbs used in moxibustion can help to reduce inflammation in the affected area, which can further reduce pain and promote healing.

Moxibustion can also be used to treat neck pain, which is often caused by muscle strain or tension. By stimulating acupoints along the neck and shoulders, moxibustion can help to relax the muscles in the area, which can reduce pain and improve mobility. Additionally, the heat and herbs used in moxibustion can help to increase blood flow to the area, which can promote healing and reduce inflammation.

Tendonitis is another common musculoskeletal issue that can be treated with moxibustion. Tendonitis is a condition that causes inflammation in the tendons, leading to pain and reduced mobility. Moxibustion can be used to reduce inflammation in the affected tendons, which can help to relieve pain and improve range of motion. Additionally, the heat and herbs used in moxibustion can help to promote healing in the affected area, which can speed up the recovery process.

Arthritis and Joint Pain

Moxibustion is a traditional Chinese medicine therapy that involves burning dried mugwort on or near specific acupuncture points on the body.

This therapy has been used for centuries in the treatment of various health conditions, including arthritis and joint pain.

Arthritis is a common condition that causes inflammation and pain in the joints. There are many different types of arthritis, but the most common forms are osteoarthritis and rheumatoid arthritis. Both of these conditions can cause significant pain, stiffness, and swelling in the joints, which can make it difficult to perform daily activities.

Moxibustion is believed to work by increasing circulation to the affected joints and promoting the flow of qi, or vital energy, in the body. This can help to reduce inflammation and relieve pain, making it a potentially effective therapy for arthritis and joint pain.

One study published in the Journal of Traditional Chinese Medicine found that moxibustion combined with acupuncture was effective in reducing pain and improving joint function in patients with knee osteoarthritis. Another study published in the same journal found that moxibustion combined with herbal medicine was effective in reducing pain and improving joint mobility in patients with rheumatoid arthritis.

In addition to its potential benefits for arthritis and joint pain, moxibustion may also be helpful in the treatment of other musculoskeletal issues, such as back pain, neck pain, and muscle stiffness. One study published in the Journal of Acupuncture and Meridian Studies found that moxibustion combined with acupuncture was effective in reducing lower back pain in patients with lumbar disc herniation.

It's important to note that while moxibustion may be a helpful therapy for arthritis and joint pain, it should not be used as a substitute for conventional medical treatment. People with arthritis and other musculoskeletal issues should always consult with a qualified healthcare provider before starting any new treatment, including moxibustion.

In addition, there are some potential risks associated with moxibustion that should be considered. One of the primary risks is burns from the burning mugwort. Careful application and monitoring of the treatment can help to minimize this risk. It's also important to note that moxibustion should not be performed on areas of the body that are inflamed, infected, or have open wounds.

Muscle Tension and Spasms

Muscle tension and spasms are common issues that affect many people, and can be caused by a variety of factors, including stress, injury, or certain medical conditions. These issues can be debilitating, affecting a person's daily life and causing discomfort and pain. While there are various treatments available for these issues, including medication, physical therapy, and massage, many people are turning to alternative therapies like moxibustion for relief. Below we will explore how moxibustion can help alleviate muscle tension and spasms, as well as its benefits, precautions, and how it is used in traditional Chinese medicine.

Moxibustion is an ancient form of therapy that involves burning dried mugwort, also known as moxa, near the skin at specific acupoints on the body. The heat generated by the burning moxa is believed to stimulate circulation and promote the flow of Qi, the life force energy that flows through the body's meridians, or energy channels. This increased circulation and Qi flow can help alleviate pain and reduce inflammation, making moxibustion an effective treatment for muscle tension and spasms.

One of the primary benefits of moxibustion for muscle tension and spasms is its ability to increase blood flow and oxygenation to the affected area. This increased blood flow can help relax tight muscles and reduce spasms, which can ultimately help alleviate pain and improve mobility. Additionally, moxibustion is believed to help release endorphins, which are natural pain-relieving chemicals produced by the body, further enhancing its ability to relieve muscle tension and spasms.

Moxibustion can also be beneficial for individuals with chronic muscle tension or spasms, as it is a non-invasive, drug-free therapy that can be used in conjunction with other treatments. This means that individuals can use moxibustion to help manage their symptoms without relying solely on medication or other more invasive therapies.

It is important to note that moxibustion should be used with caution and under the guidance of a trained practitioner. Moxibustion can cause burns if not used correctly, and individuals with certain medical conditions, such as diabetes or skin conditions, should avoid the therapy altogether. Additionally, pregnant women should consult with their healthcare provider before using moxibustion.

Moxibustion is commonly used in traditional Chinese medicine (TCM) to treat a variety of ailments, including muscle tension and spasms. In TCM, muscle tension and spasms are often seen as a result of an imbalance in the body's Qi, or life force energy. By applying moxibustion to specific acupoints on the body, a trained practitioner can help balance the body's Qi, allowing it to flow freely and reducing muscle tension and spasms.

Moxibustion can be used in conjunction with other TCM therapies, including acupuncture, herbal medicine, and massage, to further enhance its effectiveness. For example, combining moxibustion with acupuncture can help improve its pain-relieving and muscle-relaxing effects.

Injuries and Recovery

Injuries can be a significant setback for individuals, whether they are professional athletes or everyday people. Pain and decreased mobility are common after an injury, and the recovery process can be lengthy and challenging. Moxibustion, a traditional Chinese medicine practice, can help in the recovery process from injuries by promoting healing and reducing pain and inflammation.

Moxibustion involves the use of a dried plant called mugwort, also known as Artemisia vulgaris, that is burned near or on the skin at specific acupoints. The heat generated by the burning mugwort stimulates the flow of blood and energy, also known as qi, in the body. This increased blood and qi flow helps to promote healing, reduce pain and inflammation, and improve overall well-being.

One common injury that can benefit from moxibustion is sprained ankles. Ankle sprains are a common injury that occurs when the ankle ligaments are stretched or torn. The resulting swelling, pain, and limited mobility can be debilitating. Moxibustion can help in the recovery process by improving blood flow and reducing inflammation. By applying moxibustion to the affected area, the heat generated by the burning mugwort can help to increase blood flow to the area, which can reduce swelling and promote healing.

Another common injury that can benefit from moxibustion is lower back pain. Lower back pain is a prevalent condition that affects people of all ages and can be caused by a variety of factors, including poor posture, muscle strain, or herniated discs. Moxibustion can help to reduce lower back pain by improving blood flow and promoting the release of endorphins, which are the body's natural painkillers. Moxibustion applied to specific acupoints can help to stimulate the body's natural healing processes and improve overall well-being.

Moxibustion can also be helpful in the recovery process after surgery. Surgery can leave the body weakened and vulnerable to infection and other complications. Moxibustion can help to strengthen the body's immune system and promote healing. By increasing blood flow and improving the body's natural healing processes, moxibustion can help to reduce the risk of infection and improve the recovery process after surgery.

In addition to helping with injuries and recovery, moxibustion can also be helpful for athletes and individuals looking to improve their overall performance. Moxibustion can help to increase circulation and oxygenation to muscles, which can improve endurance and speed up recovery time after workouts. By improving overall physical well-being, moxibustion can help individuals perform at their best and achieve their fitness goals.

It is important to note that while moxibustion can be helpful in the recovery process from injuries, it is not a substitute for medical treatment. It is essential to seek medical attention for any significant injury or medical condition. Moxibustion can be used in conjunction with medical treatment to promote healing and improve overall well-being.

Chapter Fifteen

Moxibustion for Aging and Longevity

Moxibustion is a traditional Chinese medicine therapy that involves burning dried mugwort on or near acupuncture points on the body. It has been used for centuries in China and other Asian countries to treat a wide range of health issues, including those related to aging and longevity. In recent years, scientific studies have begun to explore the potential benefits of moxibustion for this purpose.

One of the primary ways that moxibustion may promote aging and longevity is through its ability to boost the immune system. As we age, our immune system becomes less effective at fighting off infections and diseases. Moxibustion has been shown to stimulate the production of white blood cells and other immune cells, helping to strengthen the immune system and improve overall health.

Another way that moxibustion may promote aging and longevity is by reducing inflammation in the body. Chronic inflammation is thought to play a role in a wide range of health problems, including heart disease, cancer, and Alzheimer's disease. Moxibustion has been shown to have anti-inflammatory effects, which may help to reduce the risk of these conditions and promote overall health and longevity.

Moxibustion may also help to promote healthy circulation and blood flow, which can be particularly important as we age. Poor circulation can contribute to a range of health problems, including cardiovascular disease, cognitive decline, and poor wound healing. By improving circulation, moxibustion may help to prevent or reduce the severity of these issues, promoting overall health and longevity.

In addition to these potential benefits, moxibustion may also help to promote healthy digestion, reduce stress and anxiety, and improve sleep quality – all of which can contribute to overall health and longevity. It is important to note, however, that while there is some evidence to support the use of moxibustion for these purposes, more research is needed to fully understand its potential benefits and how best to use it as part of an overall approach to aging and longevity.

If you are interested in exploring the potential benefits of moxibustion for aging and longevity, it is important to work with a qualified practitioner who can guide you in the proper use of this therapy. They can help you to identify the most effective acupuncture points to target, determine the appropriate frequency and duration of treatment, and ensure that you are using moxibustion safely and effectively.

In addition to working with a practitioner, there are a number of things you can do to promote healthy aging and longevity. These include maintaining a healthy diet and exercise routine, getting enough sleep, managing stress, and avoiding harmful habits such as smoking and excessive alcohol consumption.

Boosting Vitality

Moxibustion is an ancient Chinese practice that has been used for centuries to promote health and wellbeing. This form of therapy involves burning dried mugwort on or near the skin to stimulate specific points on the body, known as acupoints. Moxibustion is known for its ability to boost vitality and promote overall wellness by balancing the body's energy or qi.

Below we will explore the benefits of moxibustion for boosting vitality and promoting a healthy and vibrant life.

Vitality is defined as the state of being strong and active, and moxibustion is an effective way to boost vitality in the body. Moxibustion helps to increase the flow of qi, which is the energy that flows through the body's meridians, or energy pathways. When qi flows freely, the body is able to function at its optimal level, leading to increased energy, vitality, and overall health.

One of the most significant benefits of moxibustion for boosting vitality is its ability to stimulate the immune system. The immune system plays a crucial role in maintaining the body's health and wellbeing, and when it is compromised, it can lead to a wide range of health problems. Moxibustion has been shown to enhance the function of the immune system by increasing the production of white blood cells and boosting the body's natural defenses against disease.

Another way in which moxibustion helps to boost vitality is by improving the body's circulation. Good circulation is essential for the delivery of oxygen and nutrients to the body's cells and tissues, and poor circulation can lead to a range of health problems, including fatigue, muscle weakness, and poor digestion. Moxibustion helps to improve circulation by dilating blood vessels and promoting the flow of blood throughout the body.

Moxibustion is also an effective way to promote the body's natural healing processes. By stimulating acupoints, moxibustion helps to activate the body's self-healing mechanisms, which can lead to faster recovery from injuries and illnesses. Moxibustion has been shown to be particularly effective for treating chronic pain and other conditions that are difficult to treat with traditional western medicine.

In addition to its physical benefits, moxibustion can also help to boost mental and emotional vitality. The practice of moxibustion can be deeply relaxing and calming, which can help to reduce stress and anxiety. When the body is in a relaxed state, it is better able to cope with the challenges of daily life and maintain a state of balance and harmony.

Moxibustion is also an effective way to promote mental clarity and focus. By improving circulation and stimulating acupoints, moxibustion helps to enhance brain function and improve cognitive abilities. This can be particularly beneficial for individuals who struggle with memory problems, concentration issues, or other cognitive impairments.

Finally, moxibustion is an effective way to promote longevity and overall health. By balancing the body's energy, moxibustion can help to prevent and treat a wide range of health problems, from chronic pain and digestive disorders to respiratory issues and skin problems. By incorporating moxibustion into a regular wellness routine, individuals can improve their overall quality of life and enjoy a greater sense of vitality and wellbeing as they age.

Supporting Cognitive Function

Moxibustion is a traditional Chinese medicine therapy that involves burning moxa, or dried mugwort, near specific points on the body to promote healing and overall wellness. While moxibustion is often used to treat physical conditions such as pain and inflammation, it can also have a positive impact on cognitive function.

One of the key ways moxibustion can support cognitive function is by reducing stress and anxiety. Chronic stress and anxiety have been shown to have negative effects on cognitive abilities such as memory and focus, and can even increase the risk of developing conditions like dementia. Moxibustion has been found to activate the parasympathetic nervous system, which helps to reduce stress and promote relaxation. This can have a positive impact on cognitive function and may even help to prevent cognitive decline over time.

Another way moxibustion can support cognitive function is by increasing blood flow to the brain. Poor blood flow to the brain can contribute to cognitive impairment and has been linked to conditions like Alzheimer's disease. Research has shown that moxibustion can increase blood flow to specific areas of the brain, including the prefrontal cortex, which is responsible for complex cognitive processes such as decision-making and planning.

Moxibustion may also help to reduce inflammation in the brain, which has been linked to cognitive decline and conditions such as Alzheimer's disease. A study published in the Journal of Neuroinflammation found that moxibustion was able to reduce inflammation and improve cognitive function in mice with induced Alzheimer's disease. While more research is needed to fully understand the impact of moxibustion on inflammation in the brain, these findings suggest that it may have potential as a complementary therapy for cognitive disorders.

In addition to these direct effects on cognitive function, moxibustion can also have a positive impact on overall health and wellness, which can in turn support cognitive function. For example, moxibustion has been found to improve sleep quality, which is essential for cognitive health. It can also help to reduce pain and inflammation throughout the body, which can improve overall quality of life and reduce the stress that can contribute to cognitive decline.

It's important to note that while moxibustion can be a safe and effective therapy for supporting cognitive function, it should always be used as a complementary therapy alongside other treatments as recommended by a qualified healthcare practitioner. It's also important to seek out a qualified and experienced practitioner who can provide proper guidance and ensure safe practice.

Maintaining Physical Strength and Flexibility

Maintaining physical strength and flexibility is crucial to overall health and wellness, particularly as we age. There are numerous ways to achieve this, including exercise, proper nutrition, and rest. However, there are also alternative therapies that can be beneficial in maintaining and enhancing physical strength and flexibility, including moxibustion.

Moxibustion is a traditional Chinese medicine therapy that involves burning dried mugwort (also known as moxa) on or near certain acupuncture points on the body. The heat generated from the burning moxa is believed to stimulate the flow of qi (pronounced "chee"), or life energy, in the body, and can be used to address a variety of health issues.

One of the ways in which moxibustion can be beneficial for maintaining physical strength and flexibility is by increasing circulation and improving joint mobility. Moxibustion is often used in the treatment of arthritis and other conditions that cause joint pain and stiffness. By increasing circulation to the affected areas and promoting the movement of qi, moxibustion can help to reduce inflammation and pain and improve range of motion in the joints.

Moxibustion can also be beneficial in preventing muscle injuries and promoting muscle recovery. It is often used by athletes and other active individuals to help prevent muscle strains and sprains, as well as to speed up recovery from these types of injuries. By increasing blood flow to the muscles and promoting the movement of qi, moxibustion can help to reduce muscle tension and promote faster healing.

In addition, moxibustion can be beneficial in improving posture and balance, which are essential to maintaining physical strength and flexibility. Poor posture and balance can lead to muscle imbalances, which can increase the risk of injury and decrease overall physical function. By promoting the flow of qi and increasing circulation to the muscles, moxibustion can help to improve posture and balance and reduce the risk of injury.

Moxibustion can also be used to address a variety of other health issues that can affect physical strength and flexibility. For example, it can be used to treat digestive issues, which can impact nutrient absorption and energy levels, and respiratory issues, which can affect oxygen intake and energy levels. By addressing these underlying health issues, moxibustion can help to improve overall physical function and vitality.

It is important to note that while moxibustion can be a helpful therapy for maintaining physical strength and flexibility, it should not be used as a substitute for proper exercise and nutrition. Regular exercise, including strength training and stretching, is essential for maintaining muscle mass and flexibility, as well as for promoting overall health and wellness. Similarly, a balanced diet that is rich in nutrients and low in processed foods is essential for providing the body with the fuel it needs to function properly.

If you are interested in incorporating moxibustion into your wellness routine, it is important to consult with a qualified practitioner who can help you determine the best course of treatment for your individual needs. A trained acupuncturist can evaluate your health history and current condition and develop a treatment plan that is tailored to your specific needs.

Chapter Sixteen

Moxibustion for Weight Management

Moxibustion is a traditional Chinese medicine technique that involves the burning of mugwort, a dried herb, on or near specific acupuncture points on the body. It is believed to stimulate the body's natural healing processes and restore balance to the body's energy flow, or qi. While moxibustion is often used to treat a wide range of conditions, it can also be used to support weight management efforts.

According to traditional Chinese medicine, weight gain can occur when the body's energy flow is blocked, leading to an accumulation of excess fat. Moxibustion can help to stimulate the body's metabolism and promote the burning of excess fat. It is believed that the heat generated by the burning mugwort can increase blood circulation and stimulate the digestive system, leading to a more efficient breakdown of fats and an increased rate of metabolism.

One study published in the Journal of Acupuncture and Meridian Studies found that moxibustion can improve weight loss outcomes in overweight and obese individuals. In the study, participants received moxibustion treatment on specific acupuncture points three times a week for 12 weeks. The researchers found that the moxibustion group had a significantly greater reduction in body weight, body mass index, and waist circumference compared to the control group.

Another study published in the Journal of Traditional Chinese Medicine found that moxibustion can help to regulate the hormones that control appetite and metabolism. The researchers found that moxibustion on specific acupuncture points led to a decrease in ghrelin, a hormone that stimulates appetite, and an increase in leptin, a hormone that signals the body to stop eating.

In addition to moxibustion, traditional Chinese medicine also includes dietary recommendations and herbal remedies to support weight management efforts. Eating a diet that is high in fiber, low in processed foods and sugar, and rich in vegetables and whole grains can help to support healthy digestion and metabolism. Herbal remedies such as ginseng, astragalus, and cinnamon can also be used to support weight loss efforts.

It is important to note that moxibustion should be used as part of a comprehensive weight management plan that includes a healthy diet and regular exercise. It should not be used as a standalone treatment for weight loss. Additionally, individuals who are pregnant, have a fever, or have certain medical conditions such as cancer or tuberculosis should not use moxibustion without consulting a qualified practitioner.

Balancing Metabolism

Moxibustion is a form of Traditional Chinese Medicine (TCM) that involves the burning of moxa, a dried herb derived from the mugwort plant, on or near specific acupuncture points on the body. While often used to address pain and inflammation, moxibustion can also be an effective therapy for balancing metabolism and promoting weight management.

According to TCM, the spleen and stomach are the primary organs responsible for digestion and metabolism. The spleen is believed to transform food into energy (qi) and the stomach breaks down food into nutrients that can be used by the body. When the spleen and stomach are not functioning optimally, metabolism can become imbalanced, leading to issues such as weight gain, fatigue, and poor digestion.

Moxibustion can help to balance metabolism by stimulating the spleen and stomach meridians and promoting healthy digestion. By increasing circulation and energy flow in these areas, moxibustion can improve the digestive process, boost metabolism, and aid in the elimination of waste and toxins from the body.

One study published in the Journal of Acupuncture and Meridian Studies found that moxibustion therapy significantly decreased body weight, body mass index (BMI), and waist circumference in overweight and obese participants. The study also found that moxibustion improved lipid metabolism and decreased levels of inflammatory markers in the body, which are associated with obesity and metabolic syndrome.

In addition to moxibustion, TCM also employs herbal remedies and dietary changes to support healthy digestion and metabolism. Herbs such as ginger, licorice, and cinnamon can help to stimulate digestion and aid in the absorption of nutrients, while also promoting weight loss. Dietary changes such as avoiding processed foods, eating smaller meals throughout the day, and incorporating more whole foods into the diet can also support healthy digestion and metabolism.

It is important to note that while moxibustion can be an effective therapy for promoting weight management, it should be used in conjunction with a healthy diet and regular exercise. Moxibustion alone is unlikely to result in significant weight loss or metabolic changes. It is also important to consult with a qualified practitioner of TCM before beginning any moxibustion therapy, as there may be contraindications or potential side effects.

In addition to its benefits for metabolism and weight management, moxibustion has also been shown to have a range of other health benefits. By promoting circulation, reducing inflammation, and balancing the body's energy systems, moxibustion can help to alleviate a wide range of health issues, including pain, stress, and anxiety.

Appetite Control and Digestive Support

Moxibustion is a traditional Chinese medicine practice that involves burning dried mugwort on or near the skin to stimulate acupoints and promote healing. In recent years, it has gained popularity as a natural therapy for appetite control and digestive support.

According to Chinese medicine, the digestive system plays a crucial role in maintaining overall health and well-being. When the digestive system is out of balance, it can lead to a range of health issues, including obesity, fatigue, and digestive disorders like irritable bowel syndrome (IBS) and acid reflux.

Moxibustion has been shown to have several potential benefits for appetite control and digestive support. Here are some ways that it can be used to promote healthy digestion:

Stimulating Acupoints

Moxibustion works by stimulating specific acupoints on the body that are associated with digestion. By targeting these points, the therapy can help to regulate the digestive system and promote healthy digestion.

For example, the acupoint known as ST36, located on the leg, is often used to improve digestion and relieve symptoms like bloating and constipation. Applying moxibustion to this point can help to stimulate the digestive system and promote healthy bowel movements.

Boosting Metabolism

Moxibustion has been shown to have a thermogenic effect, meaning that it can increase the body's metabolic rate and help to burn calories. This can be especially helpful for people who are trying to lose weight or maintain a healthy weight.

In one study, moxibustion was found to significantly increase metabolic rate in overweight and obese women. The researchers concluded that moxibustion could be a useful therapy for weight management.

Regulating Appetite

Moxibustion has also been shown to help regulate appetite by affecting hormones like ghrelin and leptin, which play a role in hunger and satiety. By regulating these hormones, moxibustion can help to reduce cravings and promote healthy eating habits.

In a study of women with obesity, moxibustion was found to significantly reduce hunger and increase feelings of fullness. The researchers concluded that moxibustion could be a useful therapy for appetite control and weight management.

Reducing Stress

Stress can have a significant impact on digestion, leading to issues like indigestion and stomach ulcers. Moxibustion has been shown to have a calming effect on the body, reducing stress and promoting relaxation.

By reducing stress, moxibustion can help to improve digestion and reduce symptoms like bloating and abdominal pain.

Treating Digestive Disorders

Moxibustion has also been used to treat a range of digestive disorders, including IBS, acid reflux, and diarrhea. By stimulating acupoints and regulating the digestive system, moxibustion can help to relieve symptoms and promote healing.

In one study, moxibustion was found to be an effective therapy for IBS, improving symptoms like abdominal pain, bloating, and constipation.

Moxibustion for Detoxification

Moxibustion is a traditional Chinese medicine technique that involves burning dried mugwort, also known as moxa, to stimulate specific acupoints on the body. The heat generated by moxibustion can penetrate deep into the skin and muscle tissue, promoting blood circulation and the flow of vital energy, or qi, throughout the body. This can have a number of benefits, including detoxification.

Detoxification is the process of removing toxins from the body. Toxins can come from a variety of sources, including pollution, food additives, and chemicals in household products. When the body is overloaded with toxins, it can lead to a range of health issues, including fatigue, digestive problems, and even chronic disease.

Moxibustion can be used as part of a detoxification program to help stimulate the body's natural detoxification processes. By improving circulation and increasing qi flow, moxibustion can help to boost the body's ability to eliminate toxins. It can also help to support the liver and kidneys, which are the body's primary detoxification organs.

One of the ways that moxibustion can support detoxification is by stimulating the acupoints along the liver and gallbladder meridians. These meridians are responsible for the flow of qi to the liver and gallbladder, which play a crucial role in detoxification. The liver is responsible for metabolizing toxins and converting them into less harmful substances that can be eliminated from the body, while the gallbladder helps to regulate the flow of bile, which aids in digestion and the elimination of toxins.

Moxibustion can also be used to stimulate acupoints along the kidney meridian. The kidneys play a critical role in the body's natural detoxification processes by filtering waste and toxins from the blood and eliminating them through urine. By stimulating the kidney meridian, moxibustion can help to support the kidneys and improve their function, thus aiding in detoxification.

In addition to stimulating specific acupoints, moxibustion can also be used to help warm and invigorate the body. This can help to stimulate the lymphatic system, which is responsible for removing toxins from the body. The lymphatic system relies on muscle movement and circulation to function properly, so anything that can help to improve circulation can also help to support the lymphatic system and aid in detoxification.

Moxibustion can be particularly helpful for individuals who are experiencing symptoms of toxicity, such as fatigue, brain fog, or digestive issues. It can also be beneficial for individuals who have been exposed to environmental toxins, such as pollution or chemicals. However, it is important to note that moxibustion should not be used as a substitute for medical treatment, and individuals with serious health issues should consult with a healthcare professional before using moxibustion for detoxification.

In addition to moxibustion, there are other natural methods that can be used to support detoxification. These include eating a healthy diet that is rich in fruits, vegetables, and whole grains, drinking plenty of water, and getting regular exercise. Herbal supplements and other natural remedies, such as detoxifying teas or essential oils, can also be used to support the body's natural detoxification processes.

Chapter Seventeen

Moxibustion for Children and Adolescents

Moxibustion, an ancient traditional Chinese medicine practice, has been used to treat a wide range of health conditions for centuries. While it is often associated with adult patients, moxibustion can also be used to improve the health and well-being of children and adolescents. Below we will explore the benefits, safety, and considerations for using moxibustion with children and adolescents.

First, it is important to understand what moxibustion is and how it works. Moxibustion involves the burning of dried mugwort (Artemisia vulgaris) on or near specific points on the body. This practice is believed to stimulate the flow of Qi (pronounced "chee"), the body's vital energy, and promote healing. Moxibustion can be performed directly on the skin or indirectly using a barrier like ginger, salt, or garlic.

Moxibustion is a safe and effective treatment for many pediatric health conditions. The World Health Organization (WHO) recognizes the benefits of moxibustion for children, including improving immune function, treating asthma, and alleviating digestive issues. Studies have also shown moxibustion to be effective in treating a variety of conditions in children, such as recurrent respiratory tract infections, diarrhea, and bedwetting.

One of the main benefits of moxibustion for children and adolescents is its ability to strengthen the immune system. Moxibustion can stimulate the production of white blood cells and increase the body's resistance to infections. This can be especially helpful for children who are susceptible to illnesses, such as those who attend school or daycare. Moxibustion has also been shown to be effective in treating asthma, which is a common condition among children. Moxibustion can help reduce the frequency and severity of asthma attacks, as well as decrease the need for medication.

Digestive issues, such as diarrhea and constipation, can also be treated with moxibustion. In traditional Chinese medicine, the digestive system is closely related to the overall health of the body. Moxibustion can improve the function of the digestive system and promote better digestion and absorption of nutrients. This can be especially beneficial for children who may have trouble with digestive issues due to food sensitivities or picky eating habits.

While moxibustion is generally safe for children and adolescents, it is important to take certain precautions. Moxibustion should only be performed by a qualified practitioner who has experience working with pediatric patients. The practitioner should also take into consideration the child's age, health status, and any medical conditions or medications they may be taking. In some cases, it may be necessary to modify the treatment or avoid certain points on the body.

It is also important to note that moxibustion may not be suitable for all children. Children with certain medical conditions, such as epilepsy, bleeding disorders, or skin conditions, may not be good candidates for moxibustion. In addition, children who are afraid of needles or fire may not be comfortable with the practice.

Common Pediatric Issues

Moxibustion, a traditional Chinese medicine therapy, is often used to treat a variety of pediatric issues. It involves the use of heat generated by burning dried mugwort herb, known as moxa, to stimulate specific points on the body. Moxibustion has been used for centuries to promote healing and balance in the body, and its use in pediatric care is gaining popularity due to its effectiveness and safety.

One common pediatric issue that can be treated with moxibustion is respiratory disorders. Children are particularly susceptible to respiratory infections and asthma, and moxibustion has been shown to be effective in improving lung function and reducing symptoms. In a study published in the Journal of Traditional Chinese Medicine, moxibustion was found to be effective in treating chronic bronchitis in children, with improvements seen in cough, sputum production, and shortness of breath.

Moxibustion can also be used to treat digestive issues in children, such as constipation and diarrhea. The stimulation of specific acupoints with moxibustion can improve the function of the digestive system, leading to improved bowel movements and a reduction in discomfort. In a study published in the Journal of Traditional Chinese Medicine, moxibustion was found to be effective in treating pediatric functional constipation, with improvements seen in stool frequency and consistency.

Another common pediatric issue that can be treated with moxibustion is skin conditions, such as eczema and hives. Moxibustion has been shown to have anti-inflammatory and immune-regulating effects, which can help to reduce inflammation and improve skin health. In a study published in the Journal of Traditional Chinese Medicine, moxibustion was found to be effective in treating pediatric eczema, with improvements seen in skin redness, itching, and scaling.

Moxibustion can also be used to treat musculoskeletal issues in children, such as growing pains and scoliosis. The heat generated by moxibustion can penetrate deep into the tissues, promoting blood circulation and reducing inflammation. In a study published in the Journal of Traditional Chinese Medicine, moxibustion was found to be effective in treating pediatric scoliosis, with improvements seen in spinal curvature and back pain.

It is important to note that moxibustion should only be performed by a trained and licensed practitioner. Children have delicate and developing bodies, and improper use of moxibustion can result in burns or other adverse effects. It is also important to consult with a pediatrician before using moxibustion to treat any health condition, as it should be used in conjunction with other appropriate medical treatments.

In addition to its effectiveness in treating specific pediatric issues, moxibustion can also be used as a preventive therapy to promote overall health and well-being in children. Regular moxibustion treatments can strengthen the immune system, improve digestion, and promote healthy growth and development.

Moxibustion for Behavioral and Emotional Challenges

Moxibustion is a traditional Chinese medicine therapy that involves the burning of dried mugwort on or near specific acupuncture points on the body. This technique has been used for centuries to treat a wide range of health conditions, including behavioral and emotional challenges. Moxibustion is believed to work by stimulating the flow of Qi, or vital energy, in the body, which can help restore balance and improve overall health and well-being.

Behavioral and emotional challenges are common issues among both children and adults, and they can have a significant impact on quality of life. These challenges can manifest in a variety of ways, including anxiety, depression, anger, and irritability. Moxibustion is one potential treatment option for these issues, and it has been found to be particularly effective in combination with other therapies, such as acupuncture, herbal medicine, and counseling.

One of the primary ways that moxibustion can help with behavioral and emotional challenges is by reducing stress and anxiety. Stress is a common trigger for many emotional and behavioral issues, and moxibustion has been found to be effective in reducing stress levels. This is because moxibustion can help regulate the nervous system, which can help promote relaxation and reduce feelings of anxiety.

Another way that moxibustion can be helpful is by improving sleep. Sleep is essential for overall health and well-being, and it plays a critical role in regulating emotions and behavior. Moxibustion has been found to be effective in improving sleep quality and reducing insomnia, which can have a positive impact on emotional and behavioral challenges.

Moxibustion may also be helpful for children and adolescents with behavioral and emotional challenges. Children and adolescents can experience a wide range of emotional and behavioral issues, including anxiety, depression, ADHD, and autism. Moxibustion has been found to be effective in treating these conditions in children and adolescents, and it is often used in combination with other therapies, such as counseling and dietary changes.

One potential benefit of moxibustion for children and adolescents is that it is a non-invasive and non-pharmacological treatment option. This can be particularly important for parents who are concerned about the potential side effects of medication or who are looking for alternative treatment options. Moxibustion is generally considered safe and has few side effects when performed by a qualified practitioner.

It is important to note that moxibustion is not a replacement for traditional medical care or counseling. Behavioral and emotional challenges can be complex issues that require a multi-faceted approach to treatment.

However, moxibustion can be a helpful complementary therapy that can be used in conjunction with other treatments to help improve emotional and behavioral health.

Safety and Adaptations for Younger Patients

Moxibustion is a traditional Chinese medicine technique that has been used for centuries to promote healing, improve health, and alleviate symptoms of various medical conditions. While it is commonly used in adults, moxibustion can also be safely and effectively used in children and adolescents. However, some precautions need to be taken to ensure its safety and effectiveness.

The first and foremost concern when it comes to moxibustion for children is safety. It is crucial to ensure that the practitioner is experienced and trained in providing moxibustion treatment to children. The practitioner should have a thorough understanding of the child's anatomy, physiology, and psychology. They should also have experience in working with children and be able to communicate effectively with them. The practitioner should follow strict hygiene practices and use sterile or disposable equipment to minimize the risk of infection.

When it comes to moxibustion treatment, children and adolescents require special adaptations to ensure their safety and comfort. The temperature and duration of moxibustion should be adjusted according to the child's age, weight, and overall health status. Children may have a lower tolerance to heat than adults, so it is essential to monitor the child's response carefully. The practitioner should also take into consideration any medical conditions or medications the child is taking, as these can affect their response to moxibustion.

Moxibustion treatment for children should always be provided under the supervision of a parent or guardian. The parent or guardian should be present throughout the treatment and be able to communicate with the practitioner. This will help the child feel more comfortable and secure during the treatment.

One of the significant advantages of moxibustion treatment for children is that it is non-invasive and does not involve the use of drugs or medication. This makes it a safe and effective alternative or complement to conventional treatments for a wide range of pediatric conditions. Some of the common pediatric issues that moxibustion can help with include:

1. Asthma: Moxibustion has been shown to reduce asthma symptoms and improve lung function in children. It can help to open the airways, reduce inflammation, and promote relaxation, making it easier for the child to breathe.

2. Digestive disorders: Moxibustion can be effective in treating various digestive disorders such as constipation, diarrhea, and abdominal pain. It works by stimulating the digestive system and promoting healthy digestion.

3. Behavioral and emotional challenges: Moxibustion can be helpful in treating behavioral and emotional challenges such as anxiety, depression, and ADHD. It can help to regulate the nervous system and promote a sense of calm and relaxation.

4. Sleep disorders: Moxibustion can be effective in treating sleep disorders such as insomnia and restless sleep. It works by regulating the body's circadian rhythm and promoting relaxation, which can improve sleep quality and duration.

5. Pain and inflammation: Moxibustion can be effective in reducing pain and inflammation in children. It works by increasing blood flow to the affected area and promoting the release of natural pain-relieving chemicals in the body.

Moxibustion can also be used to support overall health and wellbeing in children. It can promote immune function, improve energy levels, and enhance cognitive function. It can be used as a preventative measure to promote healthy growth and development in children.

Chapter Eighteen

Moxibustion for Athletes

Moxibustion, a traditional Chinese medicine technique, has been used for centuries to treat a wide range of conditions, including musculoskeletal issues. Athletes, in particular, can benefit from the healing properties of moxibustion to improve performance, prevent injuries, and speed up recovery.

Moxibustion involves the burning of dried mugwort herb on specific acupuncture points on the body. The heat generated by the burning herb penetrates deep into the tissues, promoting blood circulation and stimulating the immune system. This leads to pain relief, reduced inflammation, and improved overall health.

One of the key benefits of moxibustion for athletes is its ability to prevent injuries. Athletes often put a lot of strain on their muscles and joints, which can lead to inflammation and microtrauma. Moxibustion can help to prevent these injuries by improving circulation, reducing inflammation, and promoting tissue repair.

Moxibustion can also be used to treat injuries that have already occurred. For example, it can be used to speed up the healing process of muscle strains, sprains, and other soft tissue injuries. The heat generated by the burning herb can help to increase blood flow to the affected area, bringing in more oxygen and nutrients to support the healing process.

In addition to its physical benefits, moxibustion can also improve mental performance. Athletes often experience stress and anxiety related to their training and competition. Moxibustion has been shown to reduce stress and anxiety by promoting relaxation and reducing the production of stress hormones.

Moxibustion can also be used to improve sleep quality, which is essential for athletes' recovery and performance. The heat generated by the burning herb can help to calm the nervous system and promote deep, restorative sleep.

When using moxibustion for athletes, it is important to work with a qualified practitioner who understands the specific needs of athletes. The practitioner should have experience working with athletes and should be able to customize the treatment plan based on the athlete's specific condition and goals.

In addition, it is important to follow proper safety precautions when using moxibustion. The burning herb can cause skin burns and should be used carefully to avoid injury. The practitioner should also be aware of any contraindications and adjust the treatment plan accordingly.

Enhancing Performance

Moxibustion is a traditional Chinese medicine technique that involves burning dried mugwort (a type of herb) on or near specific points on the body to stimulate healing and promote balance. It has been used for centuries to treat a wide range of conditions, including pain, digestive issues, and emotional imbalances. In recent years, there has been growing interest in the use of moxibustion to enhance athletic performance and support recovery.

Moxibustion is thought to work by stimulating the flow of qi (pronounced "chee"), or vital energy, throughout the body. When qi is flowing freely, the body is in a state of balance and health. When qi is blocked or stagnant, it can lead to pain, illness, and other imbalances.

Athletes often experience physical and mental stressors that can disrupt the flow of qi and hinder their performance. Common issues include muscle strains, joint pain, fatigue, and anxiety. Moxibustion can help to address these issues by promoting circulation, reducing inflammation, and calming the nervous system.

One of the key benefits of moxibustion for athletes is its ability to relieve pain and inflammation. Inflammation is a natural response to tissue damage or stress, but when it becomes chronic, it can impede healing and lead to long-term damage. Moxibustion can help to reduce inflammation by increasing blood flow to the affected area and promoting the release of anti-inflammatory cytokines.

Moxibustion can also help to improve flexibility and range of motion, which are important for athletes who need to move quickly and perform complex movements. By promoting circulation and relaxing the muscles, moxibustion can help to loosen tight muscles and improve joint mobility. This can help athletes to move more efficiently and with less risk of injury.

In addition to physical benefits, moxibustion can also help to support mental and emotional health. Athletes often face high levels of stress and anxiety, which can hinder their performance and lead to burnout. Moxibustion can help to promote relaxation and reduce stress by calming the nervous system and promoting the release of endorphins, the body's natural painkillers.

It is important to note that moxibustion should not be used as a substitute for conventional medical care. Athletes with serious injuries or medical conditions should consult with a qualified healthcare professional before using moxibustion or any other complementary therapy.

When using moxibustion for athletic performance, it is important to work with a qualified practitioner who has experience working with athletes. They will be able to tailor the treatment to your specific needs and help you achieve your performance goals. It is also important to follow any safety guidelines and precautions recommended by your practitioner.

Recovery and Injury Prevention

Moxibustion is an ancient healing technique used in traditional Chinese medicine that involves burning the herb mugwort over specific acupoints on the body. It is believed that moxibustion can help with a range of health issues, including musculoskeletal injuries, pain management, digestive disorders, and more. One area where moxibustion has gained popularity is in sports medicine, particularly among athletes looking to enhance their performance and prevent injuries.

Moxibustion can be used in a variety of ways to support athletes in their training and recovery. One of the primary benefits of moxibustion is its ability to increase circulation, which can help to speed up recovery time after strenuous exercise. By increasing circulation to the muscles, joints, and tendons, moxibustion can also help to reduce inflammation and promote healing.

In addition to aiding in recovery, moxibustion can also be used to prevent injuries. Athletes who engage in high-impact sports or repetitive movements may be at risk for overuse injuries, such as tendinitis or stress fractures. Moxibustion can be used to strengthen the affected area and promote healing, helping to prevent further injury.

Another benefit of moxibustion for athletes is its ability to enhance performance. By increasing circulation and promoting relaxation, moxibustion can help athletes to feel more energized and focused. It can also help to reduce stress and anxiety, allowing athletes to perform at their best.

When using moxibustion for athletes, it is important to take certain precautions to ensure safety and effectiveness. First, it is important to work with a qualified practitioner who is experienced in working with athletes. They can help to identify the most effective acupoints to use for specific injuries or performance goals.

It is also important to be aware of any contraindications or precautions for using moxibustion. For example, moxibustion should not be used on areas of the body that are swollen, red, or inflamed. It should also not be used on areas of the body that are sensitive to heat, such as the face or genitals.

In terms of technique, there are a few different ways that moxibustion can be used for athletes. One common method is direct moxibustion, where a small piece of moxa is placed directly on the skin over the affected area. This can be particularly effective for injuries or chronic pain. Another method is indirect moxibustion, where the moxa is held above the skin using a special device or a rolled-up piece of ginger. This method is often used for more general health and wellness purposes.

Mental Focus and Resilience

Moxibustion, a traditional Chinese medicine practice that involves burning an herb called moxa, has been gaining popularity among athletes for its potential benefits in enhancing mental focus and resilience. This therapy is believed to stimulate specific acupoints in the body, promoting the flow of Qi, or energy, and restoring balance to the body.

The physical demands of athletic training and competition can take a toll on an athlete's mental health and focus. Athletes may experience stress, anxiety, and fatigue, which can negatively impact their performance. Moxibustion has been found to have a calming effect on the mind, promoting relaxation and reducing stress and anxiety levels.

In a study published in the Journal of Traditional Chinese Medicine, moxibustion was found to significantly reduce anxiety levels in athletes. The study involved a group of male athletes who received moxibustion treatment twice a week for six weeks. The results showed that the athletes experienced a significant reduction in anxiety levels, compared to a control group that did not receive moxibustion treatment.

Moxibustion has also been found to improve mental resilience in athletes. Mental resilience refers to an individual's ability to cope with stress, adapt to change, and bounce back from setbacks. In a study published in the Journal of Acupuncture and Meridian Studies, moxibustion was found to improve mental resilience in female athletes. The study involved a group of female volleyball players who received moxibustion treatment twice a week for eight weeks. The results showed that the athletes had a significant improvement in mental resilience, compared to a control group that did not receive moxibustion treatment.

Aside from its benefits in mental health and focus, moxibustion has also been found to help athletes in injury prevention and recovery. Injuries are a common occurrence in sports, and they can be debilitating for athletes. Moxibustion has been found to promote blood circulation, reduce inflammation, and accelerate healing in injured tissues. This therapy has been used to treat a wide range of sports-related injuries, including sprains, strains, and contusions.

In a study published in the Journal of Sports Science and Medicine, moxibustion was found to accelerate the healing of ankle sprains in athletes. The study involved a group of male athletes who received moxibustion treatment for ten days, twice a day. The results showed that the athletes experienced a significant improvement in ankle function and a faster recovery time, compared to a control group that did not receive moxibustion treatment.

Moxibustion can also be used to help athletes recover from muscle soreness and fatigue. After an intense workout or competition, athletes may experience muscle soreness and fatigue, which can affect their performance in subsequent events. Moxibustion has been found to promote blood circulation and reduce inflammation, which can help relieve muscle soreness and fatigue.

In a study published in the Journal of Alternative and Complementary Medicine, moxibustion was found to be effective in relieving muscle soreness and fatigue in athletes. The study involved a group of male athletes who received moxibustion treatment twice a week for four weeks. The results showed that the athletes experienced a significant reduction in muscle soreness and fatigue, compared to a control group that did not receive moxibustion treatment.

Chapter Nineteen

Moxibustion for Self-Care

Moxibustion is a traditional Chinese medicine therapy that has been used for centuries. It involves the burning of mugwort, a small spongy herb, on or near specific acupuncture points on the body. This heat therapy has been used for various physical and emotional ailments, and it is also a great form of self-care that can be done at home.

Moxibustion for self-care is becoming increasingly popular as people are seeking natural remedies to maintain and improve their health. This practice can help boost the immune system, reduce stress and anxiety, improve sleep, and alleviate pain and inflammation.

One of the main benefits of moxibustion is its ability to stimulate the immune system. The heat produced by burning mugwort helps increase blood circulation and the flow of qi, or life force energy, throughout the body. This helps to strengthen the immune system, making it more capable of fighting off infections and illnesses.

Moxibustion can also be used to reduce stress and anxiety. The heat produced by burning mugwort can help relax the body and calm the mind, reducing feelings of stress and anxiety. This is especially helpful for those who suffer from chronic stress, which can lead to a variety of physical and emotional health problems.

In addition to reducing stress and anxiety, moxibustion can also improve sleep. Many people suffer from sleep disturbances due to stress, anxiety, or other health problems. Moxibustion can help calm the mind and relax the body, making it easier to fall asleep and stay asleep throughout the night.

Moxibustion can also be used to alleviate pain and inflammation. The heat produced by burning mugwort can help increase blood circulation and reduce inflammation, which can help relieve pain caused by conditions such as arthritis, fibromyalgia, and muscle strains.

While moxibustion is generally safe, it is important to take certain precautions when using it for self-care. First, it is important to make sure that you are using high-quality mugwort that is free from toxins and impurities. It is also important to follow the instructions carefully and to avoid using too much heat, which can cause burns or other injuries.

In addition to these safety precautions, there are several other things to keep in mind when using moxibustion for self-care. First, it is important to consult with a healthcare professional before starting any new self-care routine, especially if you have any pre-existing health conditions or are taking medication. It is also important to start slowly and gradually increase the frequency and intensity of your moxibustion sessions as your body becomes accustomed to the therapy.

Home Moxibustion Techniques

Moxibustion is an ancient form of traditional Chinese medicine that involves burning dried mugwort on specific points on the body. It is believed to stimulate circulation, boost the immune system, and promote healing. While traditionally practiced by trained acupuncturists, it is becoming increasingly popular for people to perform moxibustion at home.

Home moxibustion techniques can be used to promote general wellness or to address specific health issues. It is important to note that while moxibustion is generally considered safe, it is important to learn proper techniques to avoid burns and other injuries.

Before attempting moxibustion at home, it is important to consult with a trained practitioner to identify the proper points on the body to target. This can be done through an initial session with an acupuncturist or through research and study of traditional Chinese medicine.

One common home moxibustion technique is direct moxibustion, which involves placing a small amount of dried mugwort on the skin and lighting it with a lighter or match. The mugwort is allowed to burn down to the skin without touching it, creating a warm sensation that is believed to promote healing. Care should be taken to avoid burning the skin or allowing the mugwort to burn for too long.

Another technique is indirect moxibustion, which involves using a moxa stick or a moxa roll. A moxa stick is a cylindrical stick of compressed mugwort that is lit on one end and held near the skin to create a warm sensation. A moxa roll is similar to a stick, but it is wrapped in paper and burned like incense, with the smoke directed toward the skin. Both techniques should be done under close supervision to avoid burns or accidental fires.

Moxibustion can also be combined with acupuncture, using small amounts of moxa on the needles to enhance the effects of the treatment. This technique is typically performed by trained acupuncturists and should not be attempted at home.

When using moxibustion at home, it is important to choose a well-ventilated area and to avoid flammable materials. Care should also be taken to avoid using moxibustion on areas of the body that are sensitive or prone to injury. Pregnant women should avoid using moxibustion without the guidance of a trained practitioner, as certain points on the body are contraindicated during pregnancy.

In addition to its physical benefits, home moxibustion can also provide a sense of relaxation and stress relief. Many people find the warmth and scent of burning mugwort to be calming and soothing. It can be a useful addition to a self-care routine for those looking to promote overall wellness and balance.

Integrating Moxibustion into Your Daily Routine

Integrating Moxibustion into Your Daily Routine

Moxibustion is a traditional Chinese medicine therapy that involves burning the herb mugwort (Artemisia vulgaris) over acupuncture points or areas of the body to promote healing and wellbeing. This therapy has been used for centuries to treat various ailments and promote overall health, and it continues to be widely used in modern times. One of the benefits of moxibustion is that it can easily be incorporated into your daily routine to support your health and wellbeing. Below we will explore the benefits of moxibustion and provide tips for integrating it into your daily routine.

The Benefits of Moxibustion

Moxibustion has many potential benefits, both physical and emotional. It can be used to:

Relieve pain and inflammation

Boost the immune system

Improve circulation

Aid in digestion and relieve gastrointestinal issues

Improve sleep quality and regulate the sleep-wake cycle

Reduce stress and anxiety

Promote relaxation and balance emotions

Increase energy levels and overall vitality

Promote healing of injuries and wounds

Support reproductive health

Improve mental clarity and focus

These benefits make moxibustion a valuable tool for promoting overall health and wellbeing.

Integrating Moxibustion into Your Daily Routine

Moxibustion can be easily integrated into your daily routine, whether you are seeking to address a specific health concern or simply looking to promote overall wellbeing. Here are some tips for incorporating moxibustion into your daily routine:

Set aside time for self-care

Integrating moxibustion into your daily routine requires making time for self-care. Set aside some time each day to focus on your health and wellbeing, whether it is first thing in the morning or before bed. This can be a great way to start or end your day on a positive note.

Choose the right time and place

Choose a time and place where you can relax and focus on your moxibustion practice. This may be in a quiet room, outdoors in a peaceful setting, or in a dedicated meditation space. Make sure you are comfortable and can fully engage in your practice without distractions.

Choose the right materials

You will need a moxa stick, a lighter or matches, and a container to catch the ash. You can purchase these materials online or from a local health store. It is important to choose high-quality materials to ensure the best possible results.

Choose the right points

Choose the acupuncture points or areas of the body that you would like to focus on. You can consult with a qualified acupuncturist or do some research to determine the most effective points for your specific health concern. You can also use a general point such as CV4 (Guan Yuan) or CV6 (Qi Hai) to promote overall wellbeing.

Practice regularly

Consistency is key when it comes to moxibustion. Aim to practice daily, or at least a few times per week, to experience the full benefits of this therapy. You may also wish to combine moxibustion with other self-care practices such as meditation, yoga, or exercise.

Building a Personal Moxibustion Practice

Moxibustion is a traditional Chinese medicine technique that involves the burning of mugwort herb over specific acupuncture points on the body. This technique has been used for centuries in China and other parts of Asia to treat various health conditions and to promote overall well-being. While moxibustion has gained popularity in recent years in the West, it can be challenging for individuals to find qualified practitioners who offer this technique. However, building a personal moxibustion practice can be a viable option for those interested in incorporating this technique into their daily routine.

To build a personal moxibustion practice, it is essential to understand the technique and its benefits fully. Moxibustion involves the burning of dried mugwort herb, commonly known as moxa, on or near specific acupuncture points. The heat generated by the burning herb stimulates the body's qi, or vital energy, promoting healing and balance within the body. This technique is believed to have a wide range of benefits, including pain relief, improved digestion, enhanced immune function, and stress reduction.

To begin building a personal moxibustion practice, one must first acquire the necessary supplies. These include high-quality moxa sticks or cones, a lighter or matches, a moxa extinguishing tool, and a comfortable and safe place to perform the technique. It is essential to use high-quality moxa products to ensure the best results and to minimize any potential risks.

Next, it is important to identify the acupuncture points that correspond to the specific health issues or concerns that one wishes to address. This can be done by consulting with a qualified practitioner or by studying acupuncture charts and texts. It is important to note that some acupuncture points may not be suitable for moxibustion, such as those located near sensitive areas, open wounds, or mucous membranes.

Before beginning the moxibustion technique, it is essential to prepare the body and the mind. This can be done through gentle stretching, meditation, or deep breathing exercises to help calm the mind and relax the body. It is also essential to ensure that the area where the moxa will be burned is clean and free from any oils, lotions, or other substances that may interfere with the technique's effectiveness.

Once the body and the mind are prepared, it is time to begin the moxibustion technique. To do this, one should hold the moxa stick or cone near the targeted acupuncture point and light it with a lighter or matches.

The moxa should be held at a distance of 1-2 centimeters from the skin, allowing the heat to penetrate the body without causing any discomfort or pain. It is important to monitor the skin closely during the process to ensure that no redness or irritation occurs.

After the moxibustion session is complete, it is essential to extinguish the moxa safely using a moxa extinguishing tool. This can be done by pressing the lit end of the moxa stick or cone into the extinguishing tool until the ember is completely extinguished. It is crucial to dispose of the used moxa safely and to avoid inhaling the smoke generated during the process.

Incorporating moxibustion into a daily routine can be a powerful tool for promoting overall health and well-being. However, it is essential to note that moxibustion is a technique that should be used with caution and under the guidance of a qualified practitioner, particularly for individuals with underlying health conditions or those who are pregnant or breast-feeding. Additionally, it is important to use high-quality moxa products and to follow safe and hygienic practices when performing the technique at home.

SD - #0049 - 140926 - C0 - 229/152/9 - PB - 9781776968107 - Matt Lamination